Fevers and Cultures

)PH

y

Radcliffe Medical Press Ltd
18 Marcham Road
Abingdon
Oxon OX14 1AA
United Kingdom

www.radcliffe-oxford.com
The Radcliffe Medical Press electronic catalogue and online ordering facility.
Direct sales to anywhere in the world.

British Library Cataloguing in Publication Data

A catalogue record for this book is available from the British Library.

ISBN 1 85775 583 9

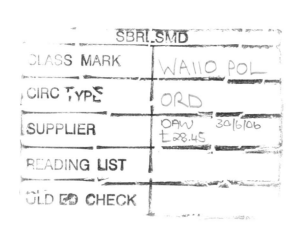
Typeset by Acorn Bookwork, Salisbury, Wiltshire
Printed and bound by TJ International Ltd, Padstow, Cornwall

Contents

Foreword

In the final third of the twentieth century it was widely believed that infectious diseases had been virtually eliminated from the industrialised world. Britain, as Shakespeare had put it in *Richard II*, was a 'fortress built by nature for herself against infection'.

The exponential increase in worldwide travel, population movements (legal or illegal), forced or voluntary urbanisation, changes in human behaviour, the collapse of public health infrastructure (e.g. in the former USSR), and antimicrobial resistance has radically altered this comfortable and self-congratulatory concept.

Conversely, 'emerging and re-emerging diseases' have become standard nomenclature in the medical literature. Indeed, the World Health Organization created a new division entitled in this way.

Novel infectious diseases such as Lassa fever, Ebola virus haemorrhagic fever, Legionnaires' disease, Lyme disease, methicillin-resistant *Staphylococcus aureus*, Human Immunodeficiency Virus (HIV) and new variant Creutzfeldt-Jakob Disease (vCJD), have combined with re-emerging diseases such as tuberculosis (multidrug-resistant in some instances) and diphtheria, to alert health authorities to the constant danger of infection and the vital importance of 'active' surveillance.

The prevention of infectious diseases has been declared a high priority in America and Europe, enhanced even further by the threat of bioterrorism.

In his book *Fevers and Cultures* – an unusual and original title – Dr Pollock compares surveillance, prevention and control in six countries, namely the USA, England, France, Poland, Malta and Uganda. The most interesting contrasts as well as common features are highlighted, and attributed to possible cultural or traditional differences in the respective countries.

The most striking examples of contrast occur in the approach to immunisation, where of the six countries studied only the UK and Uganda have voluntary arrangements. The other four depend in part or totally on legal requirements. The Polish approach is particularly interesting as it is 'obligatory' but not 'compulsory'; the former implying a duty to the community, the final decision remaining with the parent nonetheless. In the USA on the other hand, 'indirect' compulsion is practised, as evidence of immunisation has to be produced before any child is allowed to enter kindergarten or school.

This book is being published at a most opportune time. Dr George Pollock's experience of over 30 years in the field of communicable diseases and public health practice is almost unrivalled, and his academic reputation unquestionable. His meticulous research in the countries which he has compared is based on specific fact-finding visits.

It is a real privilege to have been invited to write the Foreword to this authoritative and interesting book.

HM Gilles
Emeritus Professor of Tropical Medicine
University of Liverpool
September 2003

Preface

During the past 20 years I have been fortunate enough to pay brief study visits to a number of countries and have become interested in the various systems for the surveillance, prevention and control of communicable diseases, differences which I thought might be rooted in the particular culture and traditions of each country. What follows represents a modest attempt to set out what have appeared to me to be the most interesting contrasts between England and five other countries, although I found that there was more common ground than I had expected. The study does not claim to be evenly balanced. England represents the central focus, with selective information from the other countries being used to highlight particular issues and problems, and to illustrate alternative approaches. The six countries, on the face of it, had the potential for contrast: England and France, near neighbours within the European Union but different in so many ways; the USA vast alongside tiny Malta; Poland only recently having emerged from the Eastern bloc; Uganda still very much part of the developing world. To have included some of the other countries studied, for example the Netherlands or Canada, would probably not have added very much to the general theme.

The structure of the book perhaps requires some explanation. Chapter 1 looks briefly at the current situation regarding emerging and re-emerging diseases. Chapter 2 sets out concepts which I found helpful to apply in looking at all six countries. Chapters 3, 4 and 5 are essentially descriptive. It is mainly in Chapter 6 that I stand back a little and try to interpret what I have found in a cultural context (admittedly an ambitious task for someone who is not a sociologist).

Trying to keep abreast of relevant developments in six countries, at a time of rapid organisational change and a volatile global political climate, is not easy. Consequently, although I have tried to present the up-to-date position, I regret any failure to achieve this.

Lastly, I recognise the limitations of an exercise of this kind and make no claim to be able to define a particular model of good practice. I hope that the text makes it clear why such an attempt would be impracticable, and perhaps even rather patronising. However, I believe that some of the ideas which I have put forward may be considered worth pursuing. Certainly doctors involved in this sphere of work should draw comfort from the evidence which makes it clear that their skills are never likely to become redundant!

George Pollock
September 2003

About the author

Following qualification at Aberdeen University in 1953, and the usual House Officer posts, I did my two years' National Service in the Royal Army Medical Corps, the first half in Germany and the second in Kenya. Before the latter posting I was allowed to spend some time at the Royal Army Medical College at Millbank to familiarise myself with the infectious diseases which I might encounter in East Africa (although this did not prevent me from misdiagnosing my first case of tick-borne typhus as measles!). A locum posting as acting Medical Officer in charge of a 50-bedded field hospital gave me a unique opportunity of dealing with tropical infections affecting the *askaris*, and also of acquiring a working knowledge of KiSwahili.

After National Service I returned to Aberdeen University for an academic year to obtain the Diploma in Public Health and, after a short spell as Resident Medical Officer at Tor-na-Dee Sanatorium in Aberdeenshire, secured public health posts of increasing seniority in London, Surrey and Stockport, eventually becoming Medical Officer of Health for Coventry (and subsequently District Medical Officer there as a result of NHS reorganisation). Coventry presented two particular advantages. Firstly, the City Council was very internationally-minded and strongly supported me with study leave when in 1967 I obtained a Council of Europe Scholarship to study local health services in Amsterdam and Utrecht, and also two years later when I was awarded an Anglo-French Bursary, jointly by the CIBA Foundation and the French Government, to carry out a similar study in Paris. Secondly, in 1981, I was allowed by the health authority to take on the honorary role of Visiting Senior Lecturer in Community Medicine at the newly formed School of Postgraduate Medical Education at the University of Warwick. From 1976–1990, I was also a member of the Medical Research Council Committee on the Development of Vaccines and Immunisation Procedures (CDVIP).

In 1983, Warwick University generously funded a research project to study the control of communicable diseases in France and this led, the following year, to an invitation to lecture at l'Université de Montréal and three years after that to a King's Fund Travelling Fellowship to report on health promotion in Quebec Province.

I retired from full-time work in 1990 and immediately thereafter took on part-time appointments as a consultant epidemiologist at the Communicable Disease Surveillance Centre (CDSC), a consultant adviser in the Public Health Division of the Department of Health and organiser of training in communicable disease control for the West Midlands Regional Health Authority (RHA). In 1991, I was sent by the RHA to the Centers for Disease Control (CDC) Atlanta to study communicable disease surveillance in the United States and, the following year, by the Department of Health to the State Department of Health in Oklahoma to examine the role of the state in communicable disease control; in that same year I became an honorary senior clinical lecturer in the Department of Public Health and Epidemiology at the University of Birmingham. In 1996, I was invited to be a visiting lecturer at the Medical School in Malta, with responsibility for the communicable diseases module in the newly-established MSc (Public Health) course there. In 2000, I was generously funded by the Wellcome Trust to study the evolution of communicable disease control in Poland and, two years later, to carry out a similar undertaking in Uganda.

Acknowledgements

It would be impossible for me to express my gratitude to all the people who, by one means or another, have facilitated the preparation of this work. A book of this kind can clearly come into being only with the participation and support of many colleagues occupying key roles in the countries concerned. Accordingly, it has been a source of considerable gratification to me (and not a little surprise) that such support was so willingly offered by such busy people.

When I began writing *Fevers and Cultures* in 2001 I had already left the service of the NHS for a decade, a period in which considerable organisational change had taken place, and therefore I had to take as much care to ascertain what was happening in England as I did in the other five countries. Because of this I am greatly indebted to Dr Iain Blair, Consultant in Communicable Disease Control (CCDC) Sandwell, Dr Madhu Bardhan, CCDC Coventry, and Dr Jeremy Hawker, West Midlands Regional Epidemiologist, for their help in keeping me informed on the implications of the changes for public health practice. Similarly, Professor Angus Nicoll, Director of the CDSC, and his colleagues, especially Dr Mike Catchpole, Dr Natasha Crowcroft and Ms Hilary Heine, kindly allowed me to keep abreast of developments in national surveillance and response, along with their participation in European and other international networking.

In the USA, I owed a great deal to Dr Patricia Quinlisk, currently State Epidemiologist of Iowa, but previously Director of Communicable Disease Control in the State of Oklahoma and President of the Council of State and Territorial Epidemiologists. Not only did she explain in detail the role of an American state in communicable disease control, she was also able to convey a wider perspective of United States' epidemiological thinking by virtue of her presidency of the national organisation. Dr Walter Orenstein, Assistant Surgeon General, was very helpful in providing me with all relevant information concerning the National Immunization Program, of which he is Director, and Dr Stephen Thacker, Assistant Surgeon General and Director of the Epidemiology Program

Office, kindly explained how CDC's national surveillance utilises a collection of linked systems and data sources. Dr Michael Gregg, Epidemiological Consultant, also gave me a great deal of valuable background information about the evolution of surveillance since the seminal contributions of Dr Alexander Langmuir.

The complexities of French organisation in this field would almost certainly have defeated me had it not been for the courteous assistance which I received from Dr Jean-Claude Desenclos, Head of the Infectious Diseases Unit at the Institut de Veille Sanitaire, and his colleagues, especially Dr Denise Antona, both of whom took infinite pains to explain the French systems and were prepared to cope with my halting attempts in their language.

In Malta, I was extremely fortunate to receive ongoing help from Dr Dennis Falzon and Dr Karen Vincenti of the Department of Public Health, and from Dr Hugo Agius Muscat, Head of Knowledge Management in the Office of the Prime Minister.

During my visits to Warsaw, not only was I offered thoughtfully arranged programmes of informative meetings by Professor Wiesław Magdzik and Dr Andrzej Zieliński of the National Institute of Hygiene, the former also personally spent a good deal of time explaining to me some of the subtleties of Polish thinking which govern attitudes to health in that country; additionally, my wife and I are grateful to him and his family for treating us with characteristically generous Polish hospitality. Additionally, I learned much from Dr Maria Korycka, Director of the local 'sanepid' in Żyrardów (and my Polish pen-friend), for patiently explaining to me the day-to-day professional realities of public health practice at the sharp end.

Lastly, I am greatly indebted to Professor Francis Omaswa, Director General for Health Services in Uganda, Dr Dennis Lwamafa, Commissioner for Health Services (National Disease Control) in the Ministry of Health, and Dr Margaret Lamunu, Epidemiologist in that Ministry, for allowing me to immerse myself in the exciting developments which are taking place in integrated disease surveillance and control in that country, and also to the last-mentioned for introducing me to the delights of Ugandan cuisine.

I also wish to take this opportunity of acknowledging the generous support of the Wellcome Trust by awarding me travel grants for my visits to Poland and Uganda.

To my wife, Moira

CHAPTER 1

The new plagues

To set this chapter in context, it is perhaps worthwhile briefly reminding oneself of some of the *old* plagues, if only to determine to what extent history may be repeating itself and to what extent there may be lessons to be learned. Although the word originally meant an affliction regarded as a sign of divine displeasure, early societies were apparently capable of recognising the concept of communicability and of taking rudimentary public health measures to protect themselves. Some of the activities may now seem a little drastic, such as Ramses II's expulsion of 90 000 Jews from Egypt for 'harboring a disgraceful disease', now considered to have been leprosy (McGrew 1985). Similarly, in *Leviticus* Chapter 13, verses 45 and 46, one finds:

> 'And the leper in whom the plague is, his clothes shall be rent and his head bare, and he shall put a covering upon his upper lip, and shall cry "unclean, unclean", all the days wherein the plague shall be in him he shall be defiled, he is unclean; he shall dwell alone; without the camp shall his habitation be.'

Clearly the principles of isolation were well-understood 2000 years before the arrival of scientific microbiology and epidemiology.

The Christian Church took this process of restriction of movement even further but in a more practical, and perhaps more humane, sense by establishing leper houses as early as the sixth century (Rosen 1958), and the protection of the community thereby obtained certainly had a bearing on Europe's reaction to the Black Death in the late Middle Ages. By that time, not only isolation of patients and their contacts, but also quarantine of shipping, were well-established public health measures, although of limited effectiveness as there was no knowledge of the role that the rat played in the chain of infection.

Similarly, even stringent quarantine measures were unable to prevent the entry of cholera into nineteenth century England, gaining access through the port of Sunderland in 1831 and spreading widely within the country, causing some 22 000 deaths within nine months. However, this manifest failure of quarantine arrangements did contribute to a major bonus, namely the setting up of a network of over 1200 local Boards of Health by Orders in Council, thereby creating what could be regarded as the English public health service in embryonic form. The duties of this early form of local public health authority included detection and isolation of cases, fumigation of dwellings and the destruction of infected material.

Other developments during the nineteenth century led to a scientific understanding of the nature of infectious diseases. Beginning with Bassi's work in Lombardy in connection with silkworm disease, and continuing with the discoveries of Pasteur and Koch, laboratory investigations rapidly led to the identification of the organisms responsible for many infections including, consecutively, anthrax, typhoid fever, leprosy, malaria, tuberculosis, cholera, diphtheria and plague. The discovery of antibiotics and the development of immunisation in the twentieth century obviously held out very real hopes for the conquest of infection. In fact, by 1970, the Secretary of State for Social Services in the UK felt able to state that infectious diseases, previously the major cause of death of people of working age, had been virtually eliminated as health problems (Department of Health and Social Security 1970).

Nevertheless, in spite of similar views having been expressed from time to time in most of the developed world, communities still seem to be prone, at the beginning of the twenty-first century, to a wide range of newly emerging and re-emerging infectious diseases. Although the media frequently portray these as exotic importations, and certainly severe acute respiratory syndrome (SARS) in 2003 meets this criterion, the fact is that conditions such as Lassa fever have in the past been extremely rare, and many of these infections have simply been taking advantage of more favourable conditions in which they can lodge in human hosts, multiply and spread. Although some of the conditions, such as human immunodeficiency virus (HIV) infection, viral hepatitis – and most recently SARS – represent global problems, individual countries have found themselves at particular risk of the re-emergence of specific infections, such as Poland having to cope with tuberculosis and diphtheria transmitted from neighbouring countries to the east. Even in the United States, in addition to major local outbreaks such as the 1993 cryptosporidiosis episode, and multistate incidents such as the outbreak caused by *E. coli* 0157:H7 in the same year, there have recently been concerns about the possibility of, for example, importation of cholera from Latin America, dengue fever from Costa Rica and diphtheria from Russia (CDC Atlanta 1994). Similarly, Malta has recently had to contend yet again with a major outbreak of brucellosis, an infection which has plagued its history for centuries. Consequently the terms 'emerging' and 're-emerging' infections are not really precise, needing interpretation and definition in relation to a particular country, and whether they are of internal origin or represent an external threat.

Emerging infectious diseases

Emerging infectious diseases have been defined as 'diseases of infec-tious origin whose incidence has increased within the past two decades or threatens to increase in the near future' (National Academy of Science's Institute of Medicine 1992). An alternative definition is that they are 'infections that have newly appeared in a population or have existed but are rapidly increasing in incidence or geographic range' (Morse 1995). It is interesting to note that both of these definitions include the word 'or', implying a lack of homogeneity. Furthermore, the mention of geography introduces a factor of profound significance; in fact there is a view that, with the exception of genetic mutation, almost all the factors responsible for emergence or re-emergence of epidemics can be classified as geographical (Smallman-Raynor and Cliff 2000). There are probably many other definitions, no doubt with overlapping elements, and so to avoid confusion, and because in any event their origins are quite different, it may be preferable to make a distinction between:

- newly emerging infectious diseases, e.g. HIV infection, new variant CJD (vCJD), SARS and
- re-emerging infectious diseases, e.g. diphtheria, tuberculosis, syphilis.

However, both categories could reasonably be regarded as 'new plagues' in that they have relatively recently affected populations unused to them.

Even among those infections considered 'newly emerging', there are some which have possibly been around for some time but have only comparatively recently been discovered. *E. coli* 0157:H7,

Campylobacter jejuni, Helicobacter pylori (associated with chronic gastritis, duodenal ulceration and gastric cancer) and hepatitis C fall into this category (Mortimer 2001).

In the light of the UK Secretary of State's comment quoted above, it is perhaps worth going back to the 1970s as, from that decade, the following represent some of the new diseases which have come to the attention of the public:

1970s	1980s	1990s
Rotaviral enteritis	HIV/Acquired	Multidrug-resistant
Cryptosporidiosis	Immunodeficiency	tuberculosis
Legionnaires' disease	Syndrome (AIDS)	New variant CJD
Campylobacter enteritis	Hepatitis C	
Lassa fever	*E. coli* 0157:H7 diarrhoea	2000s
Ebola virus	Toxic shock syndrome	Severe acute respiratory
haemorrhagic fever	Lyme disease	syndrome (SARS)
	Methicillin-resistant	
	Staphylococcus aureus	
	(MRSA) infection	

1973

Rotavirus was first diagnosed by electron microscopy in the USA and has been shown to be the most common diarrhoeal pathogen in children worldwide, in both developed and developing countries; in fact, it infects nearly all children between 3–5 years of age causing about one third of diarrhoea-related admissions to hospital (Parashar *et al.* 1998). A vaccine has been licensed for use in the USA. The condition was first reported in the UK in February 1979, when a 60-year-old woman was admitted to a London hospital. Two days after admission she and another female patient developed diarrhoea and over the following three days a nurse and two more patients had similar symptoms. Electron microscopy revealed large numbers of rotavirus particles. Over the next two weeks, 11 patients, two nurses and a member of the medical staff were also affected.

1976

Cryptosporidiosis has emerged over the past 25 years as a major cause of diarrhoeal disease in humans and young animals. It is caused by infection with the protozoan parasite *Cryptosporidium parvum* which can be found in the faeces of humans, and farm and pet animals. It was first recognised as a cause of human illness in the USA especially among the immunocompromised and therefore, from 1982 onwards, among HIV-infected persons in whom it can produce profuse diarrhoea, possibly leading to death by dehydration. Important routes of infection include transmission from animals to humans, especially from farm animals to young children, and from person to person. It has also emerged as a cause of water-borne infection; for example a massive outbreak in Wisconsin in 1993 affected over 400 000 people, of whom about 4 400 had to be admitted to hospital. A similar, although rather less dramatic, outbreak occurred in the North Thames area of England in 1997 with 345 cases. In fact, in the 10 years from 1988–1998 25 outbreaks occurred in the UK affecting over 3000 people (although the Government had set up an expert group chaired by Sir John Badenoch in 1989 to advise on prevention and control measures).

Legionnaires' disease, a specific form of pneumonia, was first recognised in the USA as a result of the following episode. A sharp outbreak of pneumonitis with high mortality (182 cases, 29 deaths) occurred in Pennsylvania over a 2–3 week period in July/ August 1976. The condition principally affected persons who had attended a convention of the American Legion (a war veterans' association) held at a particular hotel in Philadelphia over the 4-day period 21–24 July. The disease did not appear to be spread from person to person and attention was focused on possible environmental causes. Eventually, the bacterium later named *Legionella* was discovered and was convincingly shown to have caused not only this outbreak (presumably having been spread by the hotel's air conditioning system or water distribution systems), but also previous respiratory disease outbreaks elsewhere in the world for which the causes had been obscure (WHO 1991).

In Europe, the condition has frequently been associated with holidays abroad. In 1973, of 252 tourists from Scotland visiting Benidorm, Spain, 86 who stayed in one hotel developed respiratory symptoms during or shortly after their holiday and three died; fluorescent antibody titres to the Legionnaires' disease bacterium were subsequently detected in four of the cases. Because of this travel-associated risk, European surveillance networking has recently proved invaluable in tracing the source of infection on epidemiological, if not always microbiological, grounds. The organism was also the cause of a serious outbreak in England in 1985, traced to a Midlands district general hospital, of such significance that it became a contributory factor, via public inquiries, to the need to carry out a national review of the public health function later that decade. More recently, in August 2002, a large outbreak in the North West of England, traced to an air-conditioning plant at an arts centre run by the Barrow-in-Furness Council, provided what an editorial in the *BMJ* referred to as a 'wake-up call to continued vigilance' with regard to the environmental measures needed to prevent this potentially fatal infection.

Lassa fever is a zoonosis with the potential for severe haemorrhage and shock, predominantly found in West Africa but several imported cases have been reported in the Western world. The first case in the UK was imported from Nigeria in 1976; the most recent case was in March 2000. Initially in the UK there was a good deal of uncertainty about the mode of transmission, and so there was considerable anxiety about risk to healthcare workers. Subsequently it transpired that, in West Africa, the main reservoir was the urine of the multimammate rat, but that person-to-person spread could occur by direct contact with the blood or urine of a patient and that sexual intercourse could also transmit the infection; accordingly, appropriate control measures were established on the basis of this evidence.

1977
Campylobacter infection, although identified as associated with children's diarrhoea as far back as 1886, was not established as a common human pathogen until the 1970s but is now known to be the commonest cause of food poisoning in many countries and of a great deal of 'travellers' diarrhoea' (Altekruse *et al.* 1999). Sporadic infection is probably the rule but common-source outbreaks occur frequently. The organism is widespread in the animal world – in cattle, poultry and pet animals, and, in many parts of the developed world, the usual source is undercooked poultry. In the UK in February 1977, a Public Health Laboratory Service (PHLS) survey of 600 random faecal samples from cases of diarrhoea revealed *Campylobacter* infection at a higher level than all other pathogens.

Ebola-Marburg diseases represent related viral haemorrhagic fevers with unknown origins and very high mortality rates. Central Africa has been mainly affected but, as in the case of Lassa fever, suspected importations in the UK have caused much alarm. The first suspected case in England was a 19-year-old man who had been working with Marburg virus at the Medical Research Establishment at Porton Down; he was treated at Coppetts Wood Isolation Hospital in London and, perhaps surprisingly, it was concluded that there was no evidence that his illness was related to his occupation.

1980
Toxic shock syndrome, a severe, occasionally life-threatening, condition with high fever, vomiting and diarrhoea, and hypotension, was first described in the United States (Hajjeh *et al.* 1999). It was noted particularly in menstruating women and was associated initially with tampon use, especially the highly absorbent variety, but later also with contraceptive diaphragms. Investigation usually demonstrated a heavy colonisation or infection with a strain of *Staphyloccus aureus* producing a particular toxin referred to as TSS toxin 1.

1982
E. coli O157:H7 has, within the past decade, become a major food-borne pathogen responsible for, *inter alia*, haemorrhagic colitis and haemolytic uraemic disease. A much publicised outbreak in South West Scotland in November and December 1996, originating in a butcher's shop, involved 496 cases with 18 deaths. In another episode, in 1997, an unexpected reservoir of infection came to light when three children who had visited a farm in school parties had to be admitted to hospital because of severe diarrhoea, two also having haemolytic uraemic syndrome. The organism was isolated from two cows and a goat paddock at the farm (Milne *et al.* 1999).

Lyme disease, an infection by *Borrelia burgdorferi*, is the most common tick-borne human disease in the Northern Hemisphere. It is associated with characteristic skin lesions, followed in due course, if untreated, by arthritis and cardiac and neurological symptoms. Although popularly associated with the North Eastern US, the condition has manifested itself in certain parts of both England and Scotland; in fact, a surveillance study carried out in England showed that the disease, while still rare, had increased more than five-fold between 1986–1992 and 1996–1998 (Smith *et al.* 2000). Deer represent an important reservoir of ticks as far as humans are concerned. A fascinating study of the disruptive effects of this condition on the relationships within a New England family can be found in John Updike's short story 'Wildlife' (Updike 1994).

1983
Acquired Immunodeficiency Syndrome (AIDS) If by 1981 there had been, as appeared to be the case, a belief that pandemics of infec-

tious disease other than influenza had been eliminated in developed countries (Detels and Breslow 1991), an unpleasant surprise awaited the US. In that year the chance observation that a number of *Pneumocystis carinii* infections in California had all occurred in homosexual men, while of considerable clinical and epidemiological interest, could hardly have been interpreted at that point as the first indication of the worldwide epidemic of AIDS. The Morbidity and Mortality Weekly Report (MMWR) produced by the Center for Disease Control (CDC) in Atlanta reported the event on 5 June 1981 simply as '*Pneumocystis* pneumonia in Los Angeles'. The responsible microbe, the human immunodeficiency virus (HIV), which produces progressive damage to the immune system, was not identified until 1983. The significance of HIV infection is, of course, that until quite recently the great majority of persons affected went on to develop AIDS. AIDS, in the absence of effective treatment, had a very high fatality rate, being associated with a variety of specific infections (including tuberculosis, *Pneumocystis carinii* pneumonia and cryptosporidiosis) and certain forms of cancer, both encouraged by the immunosuppression.

Because of its original associations in the US and subsequently Europe, the term 'gay plague' was used a good deal by the media in the middle 1980s but, in due course and taking a *global* perspective, heterosexual intercourse has been shown to be the principal mode of spread, a situation clarified initially by careful research in East Africa (Iliffe 1998). The receipt of blood or blood products in therapeutic situations or the sharing of contaminated syringes and needles by injecting drug misusers represent the other main methods of transmission; additionally the virus can be passed from mother to child *in utero* and also by breast-feeding. The first case of AIDS in the UK was in 1983, a 20-year-old Cardiff man suffering from haemophilia.

The geographical spread of HIV infection is thought to have involved travel from Central Africa to Haiti (Smallman-Raynor *et al.* 1992). Some African authorities dispute this, whereas others have acknowledged that AIDS probably existed as a rare disease in equatorial Africa by 1959 or perhaps for some decades before that (Nahmias *et al.* 1986). Subsequent transmission is considered to have been from Haiti to the USA, Latin America and Europe. Although AIDS first came to light in the USA and, soon afterwards, Europe, HIV infection has comparatively rapidly become a global problem making its greatest impact in the developing world, significantly lowering life expectancy especially in Africa. In the latter continent, not only does the cost of antiretroviral drugs present serious problems but also there appears to have developed a 'condom gap' by which public discussions on priorities for expenditure seem to pay insufficient attention to this cheap and cost-effective method of prevention and control (Shelton and Johnston 2001); this 'condom gap', however, as is described later, does *not* apply to Uganda. Despite their efficacy, psychological, social, religious and cultural factors continue to constitute additional barriers to their use (Benagiano *et al.* 2000).

In sharp contrast to the developing world, the position in the UK and other developed countries has been considerably modified by multiple antiretroviral therapy introduced during the past five years.

1989

Hepatitis C, a blood-borne viral infection (only a decade ago, included as one of the forms of viral hepatitis known as 'non-A non-B') is spread principally by contaminated blood or blood products. Depending on the individual country, transmission can be by injecting drug misuse, as in the UK, or by failure to provide completely sterile syringes and needles in healthcare settings, as *previously* in Poland. It is estimated that in the USA there are around 36 000 new infections per year; this makes hepatitis C the most common blood-borne infection in that country (Alter *et al.* 1999). The significance of the condition is that about two thirds of cases develop a chronic infection and approximately half of these go on to develop cirrhosis or hepatoma, perhaps after many years.

MRSA infection, although emerging in the 1960s, was prevented from becoming a significant problem at that time by the introduction of gentamicin. However, by the 1980s, MRSA resistant also to this latter antibiotic emerged. The problem is essentially one of hospital cross-infection and therefore is best tackled by a combination of strict infection control procedures, identification and treatment of carriers, and the encouragement of doctors to use narrow-spectrum antibiotics for simple staphyloccal infections.

1996

New variant Creutzfeldt-Jakob disease (vCJD)   Although 'classic' CJD affecting middle-aged and older persons had been recognised for many years, the identification of bovine spongiform encephalopathy (BSE) in UK cattle in November 1986 led to the setting up of the National CJD Surveillance Unit in Edinburgh in 1990 because of fears that BSE might have been transmitted to humans. The basis for this concern was that if the scrapie agent (derived from sheep) present in meat and bone meal fed to cattle could lead to BSE in the latter, then spread to humans by meat consumption could not be ruled out, given that when a strain crosses a species barrier the manner of its spread in the new host becomes unpredictable (Kimberlin and Walker 1989). Although a ban on feeding meat and bone meal to cattle was introduced in 1988, cases of BSE continued to increase until they peaked in 1992.

Despite measures taken to protect the public, including banning the use of certain specified bovine offal for human consumption, the first cases of an apparently new variant form of CJD were reported by the CJD Surveillance Unit in April 1996; 12 cases had been confirmed in the UK by the end of June of that year. These cases, referred to as new variant CJD or vCJD, differed from 'classic' CJD in that much younger patients were involved and the disease ran a more protracted course. An advisory committee to the Government at that time gave as its view that the most likely explanation was that these cases were linked to BSE before the introduction of the ban on feeding of suspect material to cattle. In July 2000, it was reported that a cluster of four confirmed cases and one probable case of vCJD had occurred in or near a village in Leicestershire since 1996; the investigation of this cluster led to the conclusion that the disease was associated with the consumption of beef purchased from small butchers whose working practices led to a high risk of meat contamination by brain tissue (Bryant and Monk 2001).

By mid-2001 the number of cases was approaching the 100 mark. At present, there are too many unknowns to predict the likely future size of the problem; the uncertainties relating to the length of the incubation period, in particular, prevent the accurate prediction of the future number of cases – estimates have ranged from fewer than 100 to hundreds of thousands of cases (Donnelly and Ferguson 1999). Recent evidence suggests that persons living in the North of England and Scotland are around twice as likely to develop the condition as those in the South. This is, perhaps, because of the greater consumption of pies and burgers made from low quality meat, mostly 'mechanically-recovered meat', the residue left on a carcase after all the quality meat has been removed (Ironside 2001).

Multidrug-resistant tuberculosis Tuberculosis is currently most effectively treated initially by a combination of at least three drugs, e.g. izoniazid, rifampicin and pyrazinamide, with a fourth such as ethambutol being added if there is any suspicion of drug resistance; subsequently, continuation treatment can consist of two drugs only. If a case receives initially only one or two drugs and/or is treated suboptimally, i.e. for an insufficient period of time, on an interrupted basis or by the use of time-expired drugs, mutation can readily lead to resistance to these drugs. The term multidrug resistance is used to describe resistance to both izoniazid and rifampicin which represent the mainstream of treatment. This causes problems not only for the clinical condition of the individual but also for the community, as the persons to whom they transmit the infection will have the same resistant strain. In the developing world, this state of affairs is often associated with poor public health infrastructure. In developed countries, poor patient compliance associated with homelessness, alcoholism and drug addiction can produce a very similar result; additionally, cases originating in high prevalence countries can add to the pool.

2003
Severe acute respiratory syndrome (SARS), a pneumonia-like infection by a new member of the coronavirus family (WHO 2003), first came to light as an outbreak of pneumonia in Guangdong province in southern China in November 2002, although it appears that it was not until February 2003, when Vietnam and Hong Kong were also affected, that the international community began to take a keen interest in what might be happening. Within a very short period cases were also reported not only from other parts of the Far East, mainly Singapore, Taiwan and Thailand, but, in addition, in Canada and the UK (in the latter, initially two persons who had very recently returned from Hong Kong and Taiwan respectively).

By the end of March 2003, when well over 1000 cases had been reported to the World Health Organization (WHO) from 13 countries (including a third imported case in the UK), it was becoming possible to come to some preliminary conclusions about the epidemiology of the condition:

- the incubation period, although usually 2–7 days, could be as long as 10 days
- transmission was generally associated with close contact with a case, and therefore mainly in family members and healthcare personnel
- the case fatality at that time appeared to be about 4% (subsequently revised upwards to about 10%).

By this time also, public health administrations had informed doctors of the relevant features of the condition and similarly travellers from affected countries were being advised to seek medical advice if they developed suggestive symptoms. Globally, by the end of June (as reported by the Health Protection Agency), around 8500 probable cases had been reported, with over 800 deaths; four probable cases in the UK had fully recovered, and the UK was continuing to participate in WHO-coordinated studies aimed at elucidating the epidemiology of the condition. (*See* Appendix 4).

Why do new infections appear?

One explanation is that the infection represents a genuinely new species, i.e. having arisen by the microbe exercising sheer opportunism in a changing environment, such as HIV, or as a result of an antimicrobial agent triggering off a series of events allowing resistant strains to emerge, e.g. gonococci and pneumococci. Additionally, a new variant may evolve by the gene segments from two strains merging to produce a new organism and cause what is essentially a new disease, e.g. antigenic shift in influenza viruses. All three of these instances lie very much within the province of the microbiologist. Another theory is that some seem to be caused by pathogens already present in the environment which, because of some changes in the latter brought about by human action, are able to turn the situation to account by finding new hosts. In this situation, the field of interest clearly spreads far beyond microbiology and epidemiology to include the realms of, for example, agriculture, forestry and civil engineering. Many new human infections, e.g. HIV, appear to have an animal origin (Myers *et al.* 1992). It is generally believed that such infections may be introduced initially in isolated rural populations and that disease emergence is observed when movements take place from rural to urban locations. The subsequent movements from small towns to cities, and from country to country, offer a likely explanation of the global spread of diseases such as HIV/AIDS.

Accordingly the following human factors can contribute to the appearance, and spread, of new infections:

- medical practice involving the widespread use of antibiotics, resulting in the emergence of resistant strains
- certain agricultural practices such as integrated pig/duck farming in the Far East; gene segments from two influenza

strains can reassort to produce a new virus; ducks are major reservoirs of influenza viruses and pigs can act as 'mixing vessels' to produce the new strains (Morse 1995)
- unsafe sexual practices, as in HIV infection
- injecting drug misuse, as in hepatitis B and C, and HIV infections
- economic development affecting the physical environment, such as deforestation and reforestation, allowing exposure to tick-borne infections such as Lyme disease
- changes in feeding of farm animals and slaughterhouse practices, such as cattle, especially calves, being fed contaminated material prepared from rendered carcases of sheep, resulting initially in bovine spongiform encephalitis and subsequently vCJD in humans
- population movements, as described above, but also including international air travel – 'The microbe that felled one child in a distant continent yesterday can reach yours today and seed a global pandemic tomorrow' (Lederberg 1994).

Why do 'old' infectious diseases reappear?

If newly emerging infectious diseases are primarily the concern of microbiologists, epidemiologists and those who intrude into or otherwise come into contact with unexplored tracts of the physical environment, then *re-emerging* infections are associated with the activities of an almost infinitely wider range of people. Most of these 'returning plagues' are brought about by the breakdown of previously well-organised public health services (or simply failure to observe good hygienic practices), population movements of various kinds, developments in technology, and changes in human behaviour with regard to sexual practices, dietary habits or drug misuse. Additionally, certain political actions during the past 30 years in the developed world have been based on the erroneous assumption that infectious diseases had been conquered; such a belief almost certainly led to a lowering of one's guard from the mid-1960s – a point made vigorously by the Vice-President of the United States, Al Gore (CDC Atlanta 1995). Clearly there is a degree of overlap between certain of these factors, and population movements (as in the case of newly emerging infections) compound all the others by carrying the infection to wider geographical areas, air travel representing the potential for the widest and most rapid transmission.

Breakdown of public health services

Established public health services of varying levels of sophistication have existed in many countries for hundreds of years, as mentioned at the beginning of this chapter. However, one of the lessons of history is that such edifices can quickly crumble under the onslaught of hostile forces. The impact of the barbarian invasions on the Roman Empire was felt not only in terms of a threat to the survival of civilisation but also as a decay of public health organisation and practice. Paradoxically, war itself can provide the stimulus for protection of public health as was seen in the UK, around the beginning of the Second World War, by the creation of the Public Health Laboratory Service (PHLS) and the introduction of both immunisation against diphtheria and food rationing to ensure equitable distribution (good nutrition being also relevant to protection against infectious diseases). Nowadays, wars tend to be responsible for epidemics rather more among refugees displaced by the hostilities, as illustrated below.

Perhaps even more striking is the extent to which the public health infrastructure of a country can crumble as a result of the collapse of an authoritarian political regime. The end of compulsory immunisation in the former USSR, for example, led *inter alia* to a major epidemic of diphtheria, not only in the Russian Federation itself but also in many other republics of the former Soviet Union. In fact it was estimated that, in the single year 1994, there were between 30 000 and 35 000 cases in the former USSR. The situation was compounded by inadequate control measures during outbreaks and shortages of vaccine and antitoxin. To focus on just one of these countries, it is a remarkable fact that in Latvia, between 1993 and 1997, the majority of hospital intensive care beds were occupied by children requiring intubation as a result of this disease (Zalite 2000).

A further major public health problem arising from the end of the Soviet Union has been the increased incidence of tuberculosis in Eastern and Central Europe. Russia has suffered the heaviest burden with a high proportion of multidrug-resistant infections, at least partly due to the erratic nature of drug supplies but also adversely affected by unemployment and poverty, in addition to those cases secondary to HIV infection. A further effect of the political and social upheavals is that, especially since 1991/92, it is estimated that 30 000 untreated cases have been discharged from Russian prisons and notified for the first time (Grzemska 2000). The potential for spread beyond the Russian borders has been considerable.

The lapse in public health protection does not have to be due to a major political upheaval; it can result simply from a lapse in hygienic precautions, whether legislative or simply those of common sense. For example, eating foodstuffs made from unpasteurised milk can result in food-borne infection. An outbreak of brucellosis in Malta in 1995/96, affecting 240 people with one death, was traced to goat's cheese prepared in this way. This episode led to widespread and rigid enforcement of *existing* public health legislation. Similarly, in 1999, 60 people in North Cumbria became ill because of infection by *E. coli* 0157 as a result of consumption of unpasteurised milk from a local farm; a Heat Treatment Order was served to prevent further cases.

Population movements

These vary enormously in both nature and extent. At the simplest level there is the drift of individuals in search of work from rural to urban areas. At the other end of the scale, during the past decade alone, one has witnessed war and civil conflict resulting in fleeing of large numbers of refugees. Additionally large numbers travel across or between many countries on religious pilgrimages. Between these extremes lies the wide range of continuous movements of individuals, families and larger groups from one country to another in the search of a better life – economic migrants, refugees and asylum-seekers. All these journeys contain the potential to spread infectious disease, especially if associated with poverty and overcrowding.

Refugees are particularly vulnerable as they are likely to have left, or been driven from, their homes at very short notice with minimal possessions such as clothes, food, water and medicines. Refugee camps may well provide comparatively little shelter and overcrowding may be compounded by insufficient access to clean water, sanitation and protection against insects. In Zaire in 1996, for example, malaria swept through refugee camps resulting in a mortality rate 60 times that of settled communities in that country. Undernourished children whose immunisations have been interrupted are at risk of death from measles, as was demonstrated in Albania and the former Yugoslav Republic of Macedonia. Paradoxically, the *return* of some Kosovan refugees to their destroyed homes in March 2000, following the cessation of hostilities, resulted in a food-borne outbreak of tularaemia; rats, having taken possession of the empty houses, had contaminated grain stocks (Dedushaj *et al.* 2000).

The *Hajj*, the annual Muslim religious pilgrimage to Mecca in Saudi Arabia, can also serve as a means of transmitting infectious disease. For example, between 20 March and 31 May 2000, 317 cases of meningococcal disease caused by *Neisseria meningitidis* among religious visitors to the *Hajj* 2000 and their contacts were reported by 14 countries to WHO (Meffre *et al.* 2000).

Unsafe sexual practices

These have been responsible recently for not only the spread of HIV and hepatitis B infections but also the re-emergence of 'older' sexually transmitted diseases. For example in Bristol, between January 1997 and May 1998, 45 new cases of early infectious syphilis were identified. None was homosexually acquired; much of the transmission occurred between people living in inner city areas and females significantly outnumbered males. More recently, in 1999, 34 new cases of infectious syphilis were reported in Manchester, compared with the usual rate of 1–2 per year; 24 of the cases were homosexual men; by April 2001 the number of cases had risen to 104 with 87% of new cases describing themselves as exclusively homosexual. Trans-frontier prostitution within Europe represents an additional dimension for the spread of sexually transmitted infections. This 'trade' is offered along the main routes crossing Eastern, Central and Western Europe, the routes used by *inter alia* the TIR (Transport International Refrigidaire) trucks; because of this, in Poland, the women are often referred to colloquially as 'tirówka' – literally, 'TIR ladies'!

Infectious diseases transmitted by foods

These have become a major concern in recent years. Developments in food technology and changes in both dietary habits and certain methods of food retailing have combined to bring about a resurgence of some food-borne infections. In 1993, in the United States, hamburgers contaminated with the bacterial pathogen *E. coli* 0157:H7 and served at a fast-food restaurant chain caused a multistate outbreak of haemorrhagic colitis and serious kidney disease, resulting in the deaths of at least four children. Similarly, *Salmonella* food poisoning has re-emerged in the UK as an important infection during the past 15 years, most of which has been attributable to *S. enteritidis* (Walford and Noah 1999).

Injecting drug misuse

This has contributed a great deal to the spread of both emerging and re-emerging blood-borne viral infections. HIV and hepatitis C infections have already been dealt with but hepatitis B, one of the oldest established blood-borne infections, has increased its rate of spread by this route.

Tuberculosis

This disease, perhaps more than any other, represents a condition whose persistence and, in many instances, re-emergence in the developed world are due to a wide range of factors. Firstly, in the 1980s, the incidence of the disease was low and as a result research interests tended to be diverted to other health issues (Darbyshire 1995). Secondly, most cases occur in defined high-risk groups which occur among the general population:

- those who have emigrated from high-prevalence countries
- HIV-infected individuals who, because of weakened immune systems, acquire the disease at an accelerated rate
- elderly persons, infected in childhood and now reactivating
- those living in deprived inner city environments with associated poverty, homelessness and perhaps alcoholism; these factors can, of course, also affect any of the above groups.

How are the various authorities responding?

In the USA, the President's Health Security Act of 1993 has addressed the need to enhance community-based public health strategies, the prevention of infectious diseases being declared a high priority; the two major outbreaks which occurred in that year, referred to earlier, have clearly added force to that message. In England, the new Health Protection Agency (described later) is to fulfil similar functions. Many other countries have also identified and acknowledged the problem by attempting to improve surveillance, while at the same time planning an increase in activities for prevention and control. There appears to be general agreement that the global nature of the threat will require international cooperation in identifying, controlling and preventing newly emerging and re-emerging infectious diseases, including the design of an international policy and legal framework to assist in keeping them in check. A good beginning has already been made by the recent development of European surveillance networks and links with the USA and WHO. The following chapters describe how these various protective procedures have been evolving in England and five other countries – the United States, France, Malta, Poland and Uganda.

Bioterrorism

This subject is too vast and complex to be dealt with in any detail in a book of this kind. However, it is perhaps convenient at this point to make brief mention of it as a kind of 'emerging threat', based mainly on microorganisms which could be deployed to cause outbreaks or even epidemics of infectious disease. Anthrax, smallpox, plague and botulism represent a few of the many diseases which could be introduced in this way. Many countries have contingency plans to deal with this threat; although many of these have a restricted circulation, most tend to be dependent on strengthening the three linked capacities of surveillance, prevention and control.

CHAPTER 2

An integrated approach

The purpose of this very brief chapter is to show how the three elements of surveillance, prevention and control should ideally operate together in an *integrated* manner if communicable disease problems are to be managed effectively. Therefore the emphasis is on the interrelationships between these activities, not all of which may be carried out by the same individual – or even by the same organisation – in any locality. For example, the Consultant in Communicable Disease Control (CCDC) in an English Primary Care Trust (PCT)* may not be the Designated Immunisation Coordinator, this role possibly being undertaken by a consultant community paediatrician of the local child health service.

Although the integrated approach is illustrated by very simple diagrams, these may usefully serve as 'transparencies' through which to view the relevant activities in the six countries studied. Inevitably these diagrams imply wide generalisations and not all six countries possess to a similar extent the same 'raw materials' of this specialised area of public health practice – general practitioners, hospital doctors, public health physicians and nurses, microbiologists, etc.

The setting out of these three elements in a particular order represents a logical sequence in which surveillance – a short-hand definition of which might be 'obtaining information for action' – precedes the other two, and the proactive nature of preventive activities sets them ahead of the reactive character of control policies and procedures. However, there is a slight paradox here as, in evolutionary terms, *exactly the reverse order has been seen.* For example, control measures were instituted with regard to recognised cases of bubonic plague centuries before preventive procedures, such as immunisation or chemoprophylaxis, could be

---

* Until 1 April 2002, this was the District Health Authority (DHA). The new situation was brought about as a result of the structural changes in the NHS following the Government's 2001 report *Shifting the Balance of Power* (DoH 2001).

offered to persons at risk, and variolation and vaccination certainly preceded any attempts at smallpox surveillance. Surveillance in the sense in which we currently use the term has arrived on the scene comparatively late. Nevertheless, the paradox having been accepted, the logical order is preserved for the purposes of this work. In any event, in England this order seems to have received approval in that it appears in the text of the Department of Health guidance on the responsibilities of the CCDC in the wake of the Acheson Committee report *Public Health in England* (HMSO 1988) on the future development of the public health function.

One slight disadvantage of this approach, given the title of the book, is that cultural factors are demonstrated *least* in surveillance and most in control measures (with prevention close behind). There are understandable reasons for this; the use of the law in controlling communicable disease reflects the culture and traditions of each nation, whereas the development of surveillance has been driven largely by the aspirations of epidemiologists who, for the most part, find networking a rewarding experience.

Some of the interrelationships between the three elements are shown in Figures 2.1–2.4.

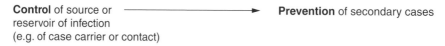

Figure 2.1 Control and prevention.

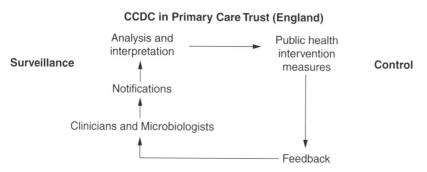

Figure 2.2 Surveillance and control.

Note: In addition to the provision of analysed material to those who have to take key decisions, feedback of information is of critical importance to those contributing the surveillance data so that they remain motivated.

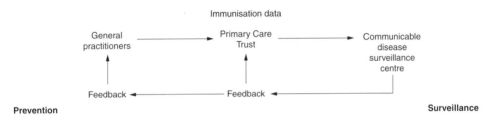

Figure 2.3   Prevention and surveillance.

Figure 2.1 shows that control and prevention represent overlapping concepts. However, in this work, prevention will be regarded as the measures taken to protect susceptible individuals (and therefore it relates mainly but not exclusively to immunisation procedures), and control as the actions taken to deal with reservoirs or sources of infection, or to cut across paths of transmission (Figure 2.4).

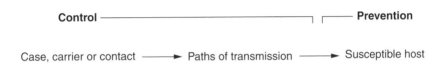

Figure 2.4   Control and prevention.

Figures 2.2 and 2.3 illustrate how surveillance not only 'keeps a weather eye', as *Roget's Thesaurus* defines the term, to signal the need for control activities, but also monitors the outcome of preventive (immunisation) programmes.

Because, historically, the development of surveillance occurred comparatively late, there has been in recent years almost a plethora of activity in the publication of papers on the subject, especially when underpinned by the applications of information technology. This has sometimes given the impression that surveillance is considered to be almost a subject in its own right, rather than an 'intelligence' base for public health action, whether strategic or operational. [The military analogy is not inappropriate. Both services require information from 'reconnaissance' sources in order to make their impact and to evaluate results.] A main theme of this work, therefore, will be that surveillance is essentially a tool to serve preventive and control activities; it cannot usefully exist in isolation. Brief mention has already been made (*see Note* under Figure 2.2) of the need to provide feedback to the data providers; this point will be re-emphasised whenever relevant as the author has frequently been made aware of the frustration experienced by these key personnel who complain of data 'disappearing into a black hole and never being seen or heard of again!'.

CHAPTER 3

Surveillance

Agreeing a working definition of surveillance is important but not necessarily straightforward as the word has had varying meanings even during the second half of the twentieth century and, additionally, different countries have tended to have their own interpretations. Until 1950, for example, in the USA (and in many other countries) the term 'surveillance' had a restricted meaning in public health practice. It was applied to the monitoring of individuals who were contacts of serious communicable diseases and who therefore needed to be closely watched for the development of the first signs of illness, but without restricting their freedom of movement, as would be the case for example in isolation or quarantine. [Interestingly, the word continues to be used in a similar manner by the military, and of course the police, in the sense of keeping watch over the actions of suspected individuals or groups (Watson 2000).]

From 1950, the term began to be applied to specific diseases and to populations rather than to single individuals, and included systematic collection of relevant data along with their constant evaluation and dissemination to all who needed to know. The first precise definition emerged 13 years later: '... the continued watchfulness over the distribution and trends of incidence through the systematic collection, consolidation and evaluation of morbidity and mortality reports and other relevant data' (Langmuir 1963). This notion has gained general acceptance, not only in the United States but also in many other countries including, for the purposes of this work, England, France, Poland, Malta and Uganda. Obviously any surveillance system should have sufficient accuracy and completeness of data, but Last (1983) has defined surveillance as 'continuous analysis, interpretation and feedback of systematically collected data, generally using methods distinguished by their practicality, uniformity and rapidity, rather than by accuracy or completeness'. More recently, in 2002, the term 'enhanced surveillance' has come into use by the English Public Health Laboratory

Service (PHLS) to denote collection of data additional to that needed for routine management and surveillance. As there is sometimes difficulty in judging the difference between routine surveillance and enhanced surveillance, in any situation of doubt ethical approval requires to be sought prior to any such development. Sometimes a distinction is made between *passive* surveillance, in which the recipient waits for the providers to report the routine data, and *active* surveillance in which special surveys are undertaken to provide a greater level of detail. This distinction, in the author's view, is not a valuable one as *all* effective surveillance is essentially active in that very careful consideration must be given to the design of the system, including the human behavioural aspects, which, it is hoped, will result in the maximum possible response in the form of clinical notifications and reporting of laboratory isolations.

Although these concepts developed most rapidly and comprehensively since 1950 in the United States, Langmuir and other American epidemiologists have made it clear that, in their view, no one had contributed as much to the development of both the basic principles and their practical applications as William Farr, the nineteenth century Compiler of Statistical Abstracts in the Registrar General's Office in London (Langmuir 1976). Farr's appointment in 1838 resulted in his taking the opportunity to develop a specific public health function by collecting relevant facts, assembling and evaluating them, and using them to support campaigns, *inter alia*, against communicable disease (Farr 1885).

The 'bare bones' of any communicable disease surveillance system, illustrated in Figures 2.2 and 2.3 (*see* pp 20–21), include the collection, analysis and interpretation of data, and feedback of information, essentially for the early detection of outbreaks, and the monitoring of both disease trends and the effectiveness of preventive/control measures. Information technology support has revolutionised the capacity of public health authorities, at both local and national levels, to receive and process surveillance data promptly and effectively in the service of prevention, control or evaluation. However, it is not beyond the bounds of possibility that the very novelty of this kind of development now presents a situation in which the sheer speed (and, to many people, the fascination) of electronic communication and information handling may lead one to overlook the basic fact that any really effective surveillance system is largely dependent on the willingness of clinicians, who constitute the sources of the data, to regard notification on clinical grounds as a high priority activity on their part. If, as a result, there is *over*dependence on laboratory reporting, valuable time may be lost before initial control measures can be instituted, even if the precise microbiological diagnosis is not known. Accordingly, the devising of methods designed to motivate clinicians to notify within the time-frame most helpful to the public health physician responsible for control and prevention is well worthwhile; examples are given in this and subsequent chapters.

The remainder of this chapter will look in some detail at the the development of surveillance in each of the six countries studied.

England

Origins

It is perhaps reasonable to consider that population surveillance of communicable diseases in England began in a rudimentary manner when John Graunt, a London haberdasher, began in 1662 to compile and publish his *Natural and Political Observations upon the Bills of Mortality*. Graunt was fascinated by what he found by examining, purely as a hobby, the figures showing the numbers of deaths in London during the previous 30 years; from 1529 these had been collected weekly at parish level, giving the cause of death as far as this could be ascertained (Clarkson 1975). He commented particularly on the greater risk of death in urban as opposed to rural localities, the variations of the death rate by seasons, and even the embarrassment which persons obviously felt about recording the incidence of syphilis:

> 'For in the aforementioned 229 250 deaths, we find not above 392 to have died of the pox. For as much as by the ordinary discourse of the world, it seems a great part of men have at one time or another had some species of this disease. I wondering why so few died of it, especially because I could not take that to be so harmless whereof so many complained very fiercely; upon enquiry I found that those who died of it out of the hospitals (especially that of the King's land and the lock in Southwark) were returned as ulcers or sores, in brief, I found that all mentioned to die of the French pox were returned by the clerks of St Giles and St Martin-in-the-fields only; which place I understand that most of the vilest and most miser-

able houses of uncleanliness were; from which I concluded that only hated persons and such whose very noses were eaten of, were reported by the searchers to have died of this too frequent malady' (Graunt 1662).

Graunt made a further useful contribution to surveillance thinking by demonstrating that *even imprecise data*, carefully interpreted, could be a source of valuable information – remarkably similar to the definition (Last 1983) quoted earlier.

If Graunt's publications might reasonably be regarded as 'pure', as opposed to applied, surveillance, then William Farr's work two centuries later, mentioned earlier, could certainly be assumed to be an early form of public health function which would not be out of place in the twenty-first century. It is perhaps not too surprising, then, that it was to Farr's work that United States epidemiologists looked in the middle of the twentieth century, when introducing a concept of population surveillance, although we have Langmuir in particular to thank for using the term in 1950 specifically to indicate the *population* dimension, as opposed to the concept of following up individuals at risk.

The 1950s

In spite of these American tributes to English endeavour, rather surprisingly the idea of national communicable disease surveillance did not *re*appear explicitly in England until the late 1950s when Dr W Charles Cockburn, the first epidemiologist appointed to the Epidemiological Research Laboratory of the PHLS, introduced a national laboratory reporting system which allowed the development of a kind of rudimentary national surveillance centre, at the time when the administrative responsibility for the PHLS was passing from the Medical Research Council (MRC) to the Ministry of Health. From the laboratory reports, Cockburn was able to provide quick feedback in the form of a single-sheet weekly summary of not only microbial isolations but also some epidemiological information (which became, in due course, the weekly Communicable Disease Report, the CDR, still published by the CDSC). Cockburn did not receive much support in these endeavours from either medical officers of health (MOH) or the medical officers of the Ministry of Health, and possibly this was a contributing factor in his decision to move to a post with WHO (Galbraith 1998).

The 1974 NHS reorganisation

The idea of national communicable disease surveillance seemed to fade until, briefly in 1968, there was a reference in a Government Green Paper on the proposed reorganisation of the NHS to the need to have *'continuous and effective surveillance of communicable disease in the community, with prompt and skilful investigation of suspicious circumstances and firm measures to prevent, limit and control the spread of disease'* (Ministry of Health 1968). However, in spite of this clear recommendation, the idea did not appear to blossom in any of the many subsequent Government publications in the run-up to the major reorganisation of the NHS in 1974, in which the post of Medical Officer of Health (MOH) was abolished as a result of the Government's belief at that time that *'infectious diseases have been virtually eliminated as health problems'* (DHSS 1970). The replacement post of Medical Officer for Environmental Health (MOEH), with minimal staff support, appeared to reflect the Government's lack of concern with communicable disease control.

The Cox Report and its aftermath

The concept of national communicable disease surveillance re-emerged, in earnest, at the beginning of 1977 with the setting up of the PHLS Communicable Disease Surveillance Centre (CDSC). The Committee of Inquiry Report on the 1973 London smallpox outbreak (the Cox Report) had, quite embarrassingly, come to the conclusion that those concerned no longer seemed to be alive to the possibility of serious communicable disease, nor to know how to communicate key information rapidly enough for effective control measures to be instituted. The report recommended the setting up of 'a highly active information and coordinating centre ... equipped with the means of rapid, accurate communication with medical officers of health', and the establishment on a regional basis of specialist epidemiologists to advise and assist in the investigation and control of communicable disease (DHSS 1974). The loss of local epidemiological expertise was made very much worse in 1974 when over 300 experienced public health doctors left the service on 31 March, taking advantage of the highly favourable financial arrangements for early retirement, and approximately 100 were appointed to purely administrative posts in the reorganised NHS (Galbraith 1977).

The realisation that a *local* public health service alone was insufficient for the control of nationally- and internationally-spread disease had come about because of the threat of epidemics during the Second World War (and had been one of the issues leading to the setting up of the PHLS in 1939). Another major factor had, in the subsequent four decades, magnified this risk, namely the very great increase in the movement of population both within the UK and between countries throughout the world. Against this background, the appearance of Lassa fever, Marburg disease and other viral haemorrhagic fevers, with the possibility of case-to-case spread, clearly reinforced the need for national surveillance.

The recommendation of the Cox committee that a national centre should be set up was accepted, and the microbiologists of the PHLS were able to persuade the Ministry of Health that it should be located at the headquarters of the PHLS and not in the Ministry itself. In January 1977, Dr N Spence Galbraith took up his appointment as Director of the centre with only one additional member of staff and a seconded senior medical officer from the Ministry of Health. The initial tasks allocated to the centre by the Ministry were national communicable disease surveillance and investigation and control of communicable disease nationally. However, when Galbraith was invited by Langmuir to visit his Epidemiology Branch at CDC Atlanta in 1977, and saw what was being achieved in the training of epidemiologists there, he added teaching and training as integral functions of the centre. An early action on Galbraith's part was to develop Cockburn's original idea of producing a weekly bulletin, the CDR, which contained not only diagnoses by laboratory isolation but also general epidemiological information from the country as a whole.

The operational value of the CDSC was soon demonstrated when, in 1978, smallpox cases occurred as a result of a laboratory infection in Birmingham. The centre sent six epidemiologists to Birmingham to help with the situation locally and at the same time established a 'control room' in the board room at the PHLS headquarters, which was able to trace contacts who had left Birmingham and arrange for their vaccination and follow-up. Later, when the Director of the Epidemiological Research Laboratory retired, the PHLS had sufficient confidence in the CDSC to transfer to it the epidemiological research functions, and the centre's functions then comprised:

- national surveillance of communicable disease
- national surveillance of immunisation programmes

- field investigation of outbreaks (but only at the request of the local MOEH)
- epidemiological research
- teaching and training (Galbraith 1998).

It was Galbraith, now Director of the (national) CDSC, who put forward proposals for *local* (i.e. district) surveillance, suggesting that each district health authority (DHA) should appoint a clinical epidemiologist who would *not* have responsibility for health service administration (he had seen that particular danger), but whose duties would include surveillance, investigation and control of disease locally (Galbraith 1981). No action was taken on these proposals at that time.

Two serious outbreaks and their consequences

In 1984 a major outbreak of *Salmonella* food poisoning with 461 cases and 19 deaths, in Stanley Royd Hospital, Wakefield, a unit for mentally ill and psychogeriatric patients, was followed by a public inquiry which was critical not only of the hospital kitchen but also of medical and nursing management, especially because of their failure to seek help from outside specialists (DHSS 1986). The result was that in 1986 the Secretary of State decided to set up the Committee of Inquiry into the Future Development of the Public Health Function, chaired by the Government's Chief Medical Officer, Sir Donald Acheson. In 1985, occurring between the food poisoning outbreak and its public inquiry, an outbreak of Legionnaires' disease originating from Stafford District General Hospital led to a report which called into question the effectiveness of the current training and experience of MOEHs in the investigation and control of outbreaks of infection (HMSO 1986).

The Acheson Committee's report, *Public Health in England* (HMSO 1988), expressed the belief that the post of MOEH had proved unsatisfactory in practice and should be abolished. The replacement post, likely to be from a background of public health medicine, medical microbiology or clinical infectious diseases, was, in due course, given the title of Consultant in Communicable Disease Control (CCDC). It was to have executive responsibility for the *surveillance*, in addition to prevention and control, of communicable disease and infection at local i.e. DHA/PCT level (Figure 3.1).

Once the concept of local surveillance had been formally intro-

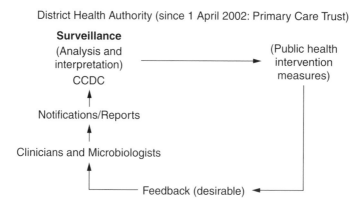

District Health Authority (since 1 April 2002: Primary Care Trust)

Figure 3.1 Communicable disease surveillance in England.

duced, it was important to monitor its implementation. Accordingly a survey of all district CCDCs (or the MOEH, where the CCDC had not yet been appointed) in England was commissioned by the Department of Health and carried out during 1990/91. Observer bias was minimised by employing a standard approach to data collection and analysis, and with all the interviews being carried out by one person (the author). It was shown *inter alia* that 91% of those in post had established some degree of local surveillance system, mostly through formal notifications from clinicians and informal (though totally reliable) reports from the local microbiology laboratory (Pollock *et al.* 1991).

The London situation

The situation in the Greater London area clearly called for special scrutiny as far as surveillance was concerned. Many people might reside in one part of London, work in another part and pursue social and recreational activities, including eating out, in a third part. Also to be considered were the vast numbers arriving daily in the capital at major airports, railway and coach terminals and the Port of London. Against this background, it was surprising to find in a survey carried out across the territory of the (then) four Thames Regional Health Authorities (RHAs) that there was, at that time, no shared surveillance database among the 22 CCDCs covering Inner and Outer London. The main reason for these problems, the survey clearly showed, was that most of the CCDCs were experiencing real difficulty in obtaining the kind of information/statistical support which would allow them to build up satisfactory surveillance databases at district level. This was particularly the case where two or more DHAs had merged, essentially for commissioning, purchasing and contracting purposes, and where (in the view of the local CCDC) the new Authority so formed appeared, to some extent, to have overlooked its 'traditional' public health responsibilities (Pollock 1993). Within a few weeks of the findings of this survey being made available to the Department of Health, the latter issued new guidance emphasising, *inter alia*, that DHAs should ensure, especially if there had been reconfiguration, that CCDCs had adequate support, including computing, to allow them to develop local surveillance and to participate in the free flow of relevant information between districts and the CDSC (DoE/DoH 1993).

The 1993 survey of the Thames regions certainly led to one important early action. The need for shared surveillance data across London having been accepted, the Pan-London Change Management Group was set up early in 1994. As a result, the London Communicable Disease Surveillance Project (LCDSP), funded jointly by the Thames regions and the Department of Health, was established in November 1994. It was based at the CDSC, to furnish CCDCs, chief environmental health officers and microbiologists in London with a surveillance resource designed to provide a uniform picture of communicable disease problems in the capital. Data collected and analysed by the unit were disseminated by the newly produced *London Communicable Disease Monitor* (subsequently renamed the *Thames Monitor*). The LCDSP was successful in getting pan-London surveillance off the ground but was eventually subsumed into the Regional Epidemiology Service contract between the NHS Executive and the Thames regions in April 1996 (Hamilton 1998).

The PHLS strategy

In order to develop a strategic framework for strengthening communicable disease surveillance for the period 1997/99, the PHLS set up in 1994 the National Surveillance Group (NSG) to commission and review protocols for the surveillance of specific infections. Five strategic goals were identified.

● To foster partnerships between professionals involved in all aspects of the prevention of infection as a basis for effective surveillance.

- To strengthen the mechanisms for communicable disease case ascertainment.
- To conduct regular and independent reviews of each surveillance system in order to audit performance against objectives, and encourage continual development.
- To promote applied research including evaluation studies related to the support and development of surveillance systems.
- To develop applications and implement advances in information technology to suit surveillance requirements with appropriate timeliness and safeguarding of confidentiality (PHLS 1997).

At the same time work was begun on the the epidemiology information technology strategy (EITS) which defined the communications infrastructure that would underpin surveillance. In recent years it has been virtually impossible to disentangle developments in communicable disease surveillance from those in information technology. A good example of this is the fact that the person most recently appointed as head of the division responsible for coordinating national surveillance systems at the CDSC has a background of biological sciences plus information technology, instead of medical epidemiology. Perhaps rather surprisingly, the application of this technology to support surveillance in England appears to have developed, as is shown later, quite independently of the other five countries studied.

National surveillance in England has continued to place most emphasis on laboratory-confirmed reports of infection. However, more recently an enhanced system drawing upon clinical information sources has been developed as an adjunct to the core laboratory-based reporting (Nicoll 2001). Since the mid-1990s, various aspects of NHS reform have encouraged moves towards a totally integrated system in which a regional epidemiologist could receive electronically not only copies of all laboratory reports but also those of all clinical notifications received by CCDCs, although the latter still also report weekly direct to the CDSC (Tocque 1999).

At the time of writing (February 2003), the implementation of EITS has included the adoption by the PHLS of *CoSurv*, a set of database modules for recording both laboratory isolates and notifications from clinicians. Isolate reports, fed into the laboratory module, are electronically transferred to the regional module (at the CDSC regional unit) and to the appropriate PCT. The reports collected at a regional level are then relayed to the CDSC at Colindale. Notifications of infectious diseases (IDs) received by the CCDC are similarly transferred electronically from the district module to

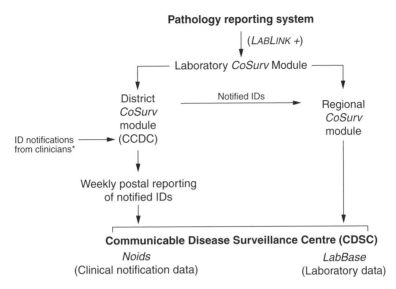

Figure 3.2 National communicable disease surveillance in England.
* The 30 infectious diseases which are formally notifiable in England are
listed in Appendix 1.

the regional module, although the CCDC continues to send these
also weekly by post to the CDSC at Colindale (Figure 3.2).

In Chapter 2 the importance of feedback was emphasised, not
only to those who need to make key decisions concerning control,
prevention or evaluation, but also to the data providers so that
they remain motivated to continue to notify (if a clinician) or
report (if a laboratory microbiologist).

At the CDSC, with new software known as *LabBase 2 **Live*** and
*LabBase 2 **Archive***, it is now possible to provide feedback in a
variety of ways, including the weekly CDR (Figure 3.3).

HIV/AIDS surveillance does not, at the time of writing (February
2003), lie within the *CoSurv* system, although it is intended that in
the future the system will be adapted to accommodate HIV
reporting. In the meantime all individuals are reported direct to
CDSC Colindale when a laboratory first confirms a specimen as
HIV-positive.

In January 2000 there was a change in the surveillance of new
diagnoses of HIV infection. Previously, surveillance relied solely on
microbiologists reporting HIV-positives identified in their laboratory, while clinicians treating persons with HIV infection were only
asked to report those who developed AIDS. The introduction of
more effective antiretroviral therapy from 1995 onwards led to a

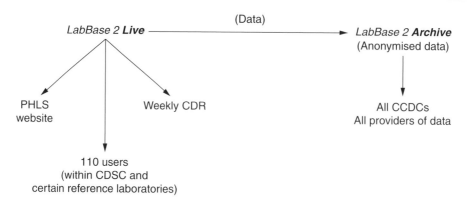

Figure 3.3 Feedback from CDSC.

rapid decline in the number of AIDS cases in those treated. In response to this change, clinicians have been asked to report all HIV-infected patients at their first diagnosis. Despite this change, laboratory reporting remains essential, not only to provide continuity with the previous 15 years of reporting but also to indicate the diagnoses for which clinicians' reports would be expected (Heine 2001).

The main objectives of HIV/AIDS surveillance are:

- monitoring the numbers of infections and their route of acquisition, thus helping to identify risk factors and their distribution, and detecting new problems promptly
- monitoring the effects of antiretroviral treatment
- increasing professional and public awareness
- informing policy-makers and service providers
- allowing comparisons with other countries.

HIV surveillance has demonstrated, for example, that of the 3550 new infections identified in the UK in the year 2000:

- 1746 were acquired heterosexually (the majority abroad, usually in sub-Saharan Africa, before coming to the UK)
- 1374 resulted from sex between men
- 94 were infected by injecting drug misuse
- 87 resulted from mother to infant transmission
- 20 occurred as a result of blood or tissue transfer.

Surveillance of other sexually transmitted diseases which, like HIV infection, are not 'notifiable' in the legalistic sense, is carried out by consultants in genitourinary medicine clinics who are required to make regular returns of the numbers of new attendances to the CDSC. As with HIV reporting, there are no data given that could identify any individual, and only in the case of syphilis and gonorrhoea does the age of the patient have to be stated. The value of this surveillance has been demonstrated by drawing attention to, for example, outbreaks of syphilis among homosexual men of the kind referred to in Chapter 1, in Manchester. This resulted in a new 'national syphilis awareness campaign' being launched in September 2001, funded by the Department of Health and implemented by the Terrence Higgins Trust with expert input from the PHLS.

United States

Origins

The United States Public Health Service (USPHS), with its Hygienic Laboratory, could be regarded as the originator of surveillance because of a variety of field studies which it mounted, and by 1933 death registration had established an early national basis for such surveillance (Langmuir 1963). Subsequently the Second World War had prompted the USPHS to try to control indigenous malaria in the Southern States, where many of the military camps were located. The programme was based in Atlanta, Georgia, and when peace returned it widened its responsibilities and in 1946 took on the title of Communicable Disease Center (CDC), later to become the Centers for Disease Control and Prevention with the same initials (Mullan 1989). With Langmuir as its chief epidemiologist, in the 1950s the scene was set for the new concept of surveillance to be developed.

All of this had been made possible by the Public Health Service Act of 1944 which specified a wider organisation for the USPHS, giving *federal* public health a new identity and status in post-war America. This represented quite an achievement as, from the signing of the Constitution, powers regarding public health (and most other 'personal' activities such as education and welfare) were left to the individual states according to 'states' rights' (Fee 1997). In the United States, the authority to require the notification of cases within any state resides in the appropriate legislature of that state. State reporting requirements also vary among diseases to be reported, time-frames for reporting, agencies receiving reports, persons required to report, and penalties for not reporting (Chorba *et al.* 1989). Although both federal and state governments have powers to protect the public's health, any surveillance system must be conducted under the aegis of the relevant state health laws or regulations in order to avoid any activities which violate such states (Thacker 1996). However, the Council of State and Territorial Epidemiologists has since 1951 determined, in conjunction with the CDC, which diseases should be reported by states to the USPHS (Thacker and Berkelman 1992), and also, on a consensus basis, which diseases should form the 'core' of the list of reportable diseases in *every* state (Quinlisk 1998).

The key influence of Langmuir

Although continuing to praise William Farr's seminal contribution to the population concept of surveillance, it was unquestionably United States epidemiologists themselves who, led by Langmuir, made the most rapid strides in this field during the second half of the twentieth century. The application of this approach had been able to demonstrate, for example:

- that simple appraisals of malaria morbidity and mortality had exaggerated the incidence of the disease and when new criteria, including laboratory studies, were adopted it was realised that malaria had disappeared as an *endemic* disease from the Southern states, probably by the mid-1940s
- how the 1955 outbreak of poliomyelitis among both those inoculated with the new (Salk) killed vaccine (79 cases, 61 paralytic) and their contacts (105 cases, 80 paralytic) could be traced to two production batches of vaccine from a single manufacturer (Cutter Laboratories), so that the general vaccination programme did not have to be abandoned, although a thorough review of *all* production and safety procedures was clearly an immediate priority (Langmuir 1963).

Some much more recent events have emphasised the essential role of public health surveillance, *and the key role of clinicians*, in alerting the relevant authorities to the risk of bioterrorism or other potentially serious outbreak. For example, in October 2001, a Florida doctor's ability to consider anthrax as a possible diagnosis and his prompt reporting of this to the local health department led not only to the involvement of the State Department of Health and CDC to assist in the investigation but also to the latter being able to warn epidemiologists throughout the nation to be particularly vigilant. This led to one of the New York City cases being correctly diagnosed, having been earlier treated for a suspected reaction to a spider bite (MMWR 2001).

There have also been many other illustrations of the value of this approach. For example, as Sencer (1995) points out in a report to WHO, during the swine influenza immunisation programme in 1976, CDC established surveillance of adverse reactions and thus was able to detect the temporal association of Guillain-Barré Syndrome with vaccine administration, leading to the discontinuation of the immunisation programme. Furthermore, the demonstration in 1980 that the development of toxic shock syndrome, referred to in Chapter 1, was associated with tampon use was facilitated by case ascertainment as part of a surveillance system (Thacker and Berkelman 1992). Additionally, surveillance for AIDS has been one of the most dynamic surveillance systems in the history of public health since its inception in June 1981 when the first cases of *Pneumocystis carinii* pneumonia were recognised in five homosexual men in Los Angeles, also referred to in Chapter 1. Lastly, in 1984, surveillance of pneumonia deaths in New York City, jointly by the City's Health Department and CDC, led to an epidemiological investigation which showed for the first time the relationship of HIV infection and tuberculosis (Sencer 1985).

In 1961, Langmuir, in his capacity as Editor of the CDC's new publication *Morbidity and Mortality Weekly Report (MMWR)*, had been able to persuade state and local health departments to use the document as a reporting system which would enhance their relationship with the CDC. He encouraged CDC staff and health officials at many levels to write articles for the *MMWR*; this practice developed their communication skills and showed them the value of disseminating information to 'those who need to know' (Thacker and Gregg 1996). (This use of the document for keeping people in the picture, especially those who were responsible for providing the data in the first instance, has been copied in many other countries and is a useful means of keeping those individuals motivated.) In addition to his constant pressure on health departments to use the *MMWR* for their own purposes, he ensured that they were properly credited for recognising and reporting the health events within their jurisdiction and for taking responsibility for such events. Even after Langmuir had retired from the CDC in 1970, his belief in the value of surveillance as a rigorous public health discipline survived in both the CDC and the public health infrastructure, although more sophisticated statistical techniques along with specially designed computer software continued to improve the capacity for analysing surveillance data (Thacker and Gregg 1996).

The applications of information technology

The United States was an early entrant into the use of electronic data processing as a means of improving surveillance although, given the independence of each state, progress could only be gradual. However, the modest beginning in 1984, with a telecommunications network linking six states (Colorado, Michigan, Minnesota, New York, Washington, Wisconsin) to CDC, the Epidemiologic Surveillance Project (ESP), represented the earliest United States' venture in transferring infectious disease data electronically to form the nucleus of a *national* computerised surveillance database (Graitcer and Burton 1987). Interestingly enough, software originally developed for use in epidemic investigations was found to be capable of being adapted within the CDC for surveillance purposes in 1987 and subsequently used in 20 states (Thacker and Berkelman 1988). By 1989 all 50 states were using computerised surveillance systems and transmitting surveillance data in a standard format to the CDC (*MMWR* 1991).

A major step forward was taken in 1991 with the introduction of the National Electronic Telecommunications System for Surveillance (NETSS), developed by the CDC and the Council of State and Territorial Epidemiologists. This allowed the collecting, transmitting, analysing and publishing of weekly reports of notifiable infectious diseases from the 50 states, New York City, the District of Columbia and certain other territories. Operation of NETSS was facilitated by professional agreements on reportable conditions, protocols for formatting and transmitting data, standard case definitions and designated staff members in each participating agency who were to provide and prepare the data for weekly publication in the *MMWR* (*MMWR* 1991).

The State of Oklahoma

The State of Oklahoma (population just over three million) can be regarded as *illustrative* for this purpose rather than representative,

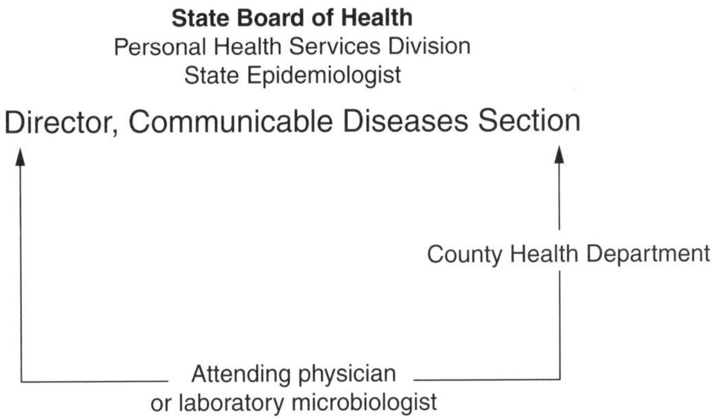

State Board of Health
Personal Health Services Division
State Epidemiologist

Director, Communicable Diseases Section

County Health Department

Attending physician
or laboratory microbiologist

Figure 3.4 Communicable disease surveillance in Oklahoma.

because of the diversity of the states in terms of size of both population and geographical area. Appendix 3 lists the diseases which are reportable in this state, those in bold letters needing to be reported promptly by telephone. Formal reporting is the responsibility of the attending physician (or microbiologist, if the diagnosis is made initially by laboratory isolation). The report is made either direct to the unit headed by the Director, Communicable Diseases Section, within the State Epidemiologist's Department or to the County Health Department covering the area in which the case has occurred. In the latter instance, the County is required to pass on the details to the State as soon as possible so that the Director has all the information required to institute whatever control measures may be considered appropriate (Figure 3.4).

A study carried out in Oklahoma showed the practical operation of the NETTS system as follows.

1 A weekly transmission file of reported conditions within the state is sent electronically to the CDC.
2 The CDC is thereafter responsible for disseminating the information, on the nation-wide situation, to all states.
3 Within the State Department of Health itself, a monthly epidemiological bulletin is prepared from the data and circulated widely to healthcare professionals and other interested personnel throughout the state. The bulletin includes information on topics which are frequently the subject of questions from not only health personnel but also school staff and parents (Pollock 1992).

[This last item is an excellent example of *one* part of what Thacker, in 1996, has called 'the human element in surveillance' in which the system has to be rendered acceptable to all who play a part in the collection, analysis, dissemination and use of the data, preferably by making personal contact whenever possible to 'humanise' what might otherwise be perceived as an impersonal activity.]

France

Origins

In France, until the 1960s, communicable disease surveillance did not *appear* to represent much cause for concern. Even in 1983, when the author raised the question with a local public health physician he received the following jocular reply: 'La surveillance des maladies transmissibles en France? Ça n'existe pas!' Obviously this was an absurd exaggeration but an indication perhaps that the topic was not seen to represent any particular priority. In fact, all formal requirements with regard to the subject are to be found in the codified system of public health law, in effect in *Art. Lois 1–18* of the *Code de la Santé Publique*. In accordance with this law, in the 1960s the required arrangements for surveillance had already been clearly set out by the Decree of January 1960 listing 30 communicable diseases which *had* to be notified and a further nine where notification was optional but still encouraged. Notification had to be made by the attending clinician to the Médecin Inspecteur de Santé Publique (MISP), the senior public health physician of the relevant Direction Départementale des Affaires Sanitaires et Sociales (DDASS), the health and social office of the département. The MISP, in turn, had to inform the medical epidemiologist staff of the Bureau des Maladies Transmissibles (BMT), the infectious diseases section of the Direction Générale de la Santé (DGS), the relevant part of the Ministère chargé de la Santé (the Ministry responsible, at any given time, for health matters) in Paris. It was accepted that surveillance was a strongly centralised activity coordinated by a group of highly specialised medical epidemiologist civil servants (Figure 3.5).

Contrary to appearances, a considerable degree of professional/governmental concern *had* been shown, for example in 1983 when the BMT of the DGS, the relevant part of the Ministry of Health in Paris, began to publish a weekly bulletin of communicable disease

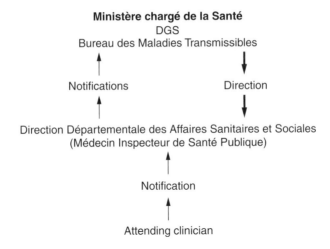

Figure 3.5 Communicable disease surveillance in France prior to 1992.
(Desenclos 1998a and b)

incidence and trends, the *Bulletin Épidémiologique Hebdomadaire
(BEH)*, as part of the process of disseminating information to
relevant professionals. However, by 1985, the BMT was already
admitting that what appeared to be a flagrant disregard by clinicians of the need to notify was leading to a considerable lack of
reliable data and the Government's intentions with regard to the
future arrangements for surveillance were given wide publicity
(Bouvet 1985). These were embodied in due course in the Decree
of 10 June 1986 and included the following.

1 A radically altered approach to compulsory notification, involving two new lists:
   - a list of 7 conditions requiring exceptional measures at
     national or international level: cholera, plague, smallpox,
     yellow fever, rabies, typhus fever, African haemorrhagic
     fevers
   - a second list of 11 conditions where action would most
     appropriately be carried out at local level: typhoid and para-
     typhoid fevers, tuberculosis, tetanus, poliomyelitis, diphtheria,
     meningococcal infections, food poisoning, botulism, non-
     imported malaria, AIDS (confirmed), brucellosis. It was felt
     that the seriousness of these conditions was unarguable and
     that clinicians would therefore be motivated to notify them,
     without fail, to the MISP.
2 A greater use of data from other sources: death certificates,

hospital returns, data from the Armed Services, National Health Insurance Fund statistics, etc.

3 The use of a new network of volunteer 'sentinel' general practitioners who were to notify by MINITEL (a videotext home server distributed free of charge by the National Telecommunications Company), initially cases of influenza-like illness, presumed viral hepatitis, measles, male urethritis and mumps; subsequently acute diarrhoea, chickenpox and HIV infection were added. Notifications were to be made to the Institut National de la Santé et de la Recherche Médicale (INSERM), a national, largely laboratory-based research organisation.

(Because of the novelty and special significance of the network, a brief note on its development follows at the end of this section, *see* p 46.)

Various Decrees followed in relation to specific issues such as the addition of imported malaria and legionellosis to the compulsorily notifiable list (1987), prophylaxis against meningococcal infection (1990), and making CJD and listeriosis notifiable (1996 and 1998, respectively).

A major reappraisal of the situation took place in 1991 setting out the following.

1 The objectives and principles of surveillance, making it clear how much had been gained from experience in the United States, especially in making a distinction between surveillance for public health practice (control measures, etc.) and surveillance for the purposes of epidemiological research.

2 The various systems in operation, including compulsory notification, the role of national reference centres, the contribution of the sentinel general practitioners, the national laboratory network and the various arrangements for carrying out specific surveys and enquiries.

3 The arrangements for disseminating information via the *BEH* (which at that time had about 5000 subscribers), while encouraging individual MISPs to produce similar epidemiological bulletins within their own départements (Hubert *et al.* 1991).

The Réseau National de Santé Publique

In 1992, a national public health network, the Réseau National de Santé Publique (RNSP), based in Paris, was created jointly by the

DGS, INSERM and the National School of Public Health, the École Nationale de Santé Publique (ENSP). Its functions were to assume overall responsibility for national epidemiological surveillance and investigation, evaluation of health risks of infectious or environmental origin, processing and analysis of epidemiological data and developing the capacity to mount any urgent investigation if the situation demanded it (Ministère du Travail et des Affaires Sociales 1996). Within the RNSP, one division, the Unité des Maladies Infectieuses (UMI), was to concern itself with communicable disease matters, while other specialised divisions dealt with specific issues, for example air and water pollution, and toxic materials in the soil (RNSP 1996).

This new and wide-ranging organisation was obviously going to have an impact on the surveillance functions of the medical epidemiologist civil servants at the BMT and in January 1996 the DGS transferred the responsibility for the operational management of the arrangements for communicable disease surveillance to the RNSP, on the understanding that it would work in close liaison with the MISPs in the various DDASSs for the purpose of both improving the quality of the data and disseminating relevant information (RNSP 1997). Hence the flow of information resulting, for example, from compulsory notifications, sentinel general practitioners, laboratory and hospital voluntary surveillance systems – RENAGO (gonorrhoea), EPiBAC (bacterial meningitis), etc. – and the national reference centres was radically changed. In addition, new surveillance tools were created following an in-depth appraisal of surveillance needs for infectious diseases carried out in 1995. These new surveillance activities (haemolytic uraemic syndrome, pertussis, hepatitis C) were implemented in the following years (Figure 3.6).

In 1996, Aquilino Morelle produced a satirical tract, *La défaite de la santé publique*, in which he described the 'three affairs of contaminated blood', namely in the treatment of haemophiliacs (HIV), blood transfusions after childbirth or surgical operations (HIV), and also contamination by hepatitis C virus (Morelle 1996). This publication also described the transmission of CJD by growth hormone which continued to be distributed for several months after the danger had been recognised. Morelle expressed the view that, five years after the discovery of these contaminations in 1991, the French public had come to the conclusion that this represented 'a veritable collapse of their system of public health'. In due course, the responsible Government officials were tried and convicted in the High Court of Justice. An official, and rather less

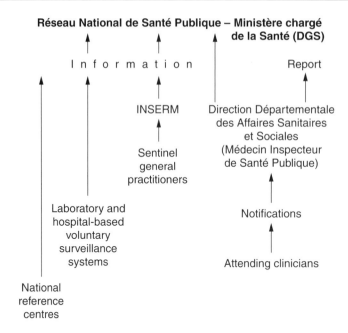

Figure 3.6 Communicable disease surveillance in France 1992–1998.

critical, account of these events is to be found in *Quand la santé devient publique* in which Jean-François Girard (1998), Director-General of Health for more than 15 years, makes the point that the outcome has been to project health matters to the forefront of the public mind, and that health is in the process of becoming the concern of everyone.

The Institut de Veille Sanitaire

It was not surprising, then, that on 1 July 1998 a further radical reorganisation of the arrangements for national surveillance occurred as a result of the promulgation of *Loi No 98-535* concerned with, among other things, the concept of 'health vigilance' – veille et alerte sanitaires. Under this law, a new national committee of health security, the Comité Nationale de la Sécurité Sanitaire, was to be charged with examining those issues which might affect the health of the nation's population, and also with coordinating the policies of a new Institute of Health Vigilance, the Institut de Veille Sanitaire (InVS). This Institute, created from the RNSP and therefore charged with overall responsibility for carrying out national communicable disease surveillance along

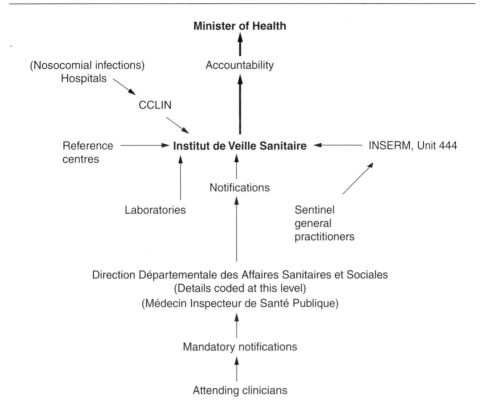

Figure 3.7   Communicable disease surveillance in France from 1998/2000 onwards.

with health risk assessment and the alerting of relevant organisations concerned with public health, was placed directly under the supervision of the Minister of Health. Additionally, new responsibilities were allocated to it in connection with antibiotic resistance and hospital-acquired infection. For the latter, a system of five inter-regional structures, Centre de Coordination Interregionale de la Lutte Contre les Infections Nosocomiales (CCLIN), had been created by the Ministry of Health in 1995. In order to organise and structure the surveillance of nosocomial infection, the InVS and the CCLINs created the Réseau d'Alerte d'Investigation et de Surveillance in 2000 (Figure 3.7).

The flow-chart (Figure 3.7) applies to the majority of notifiable infectious diseases. Special arrangements apply in the case of certain infections such as HIV and hepatitis B, in which the laboratory, after coding the details, informs both the DDASS and the attending clinician simultaneously; legionellosis, in which the

European Working Group on Legionella Infection (EWGLI) plays a key part in determining if the infection has affected more than one European country; and listeriosis, in which the relevant National Reference Centre has an important role (Desenclos 2001).

Special note on the sentinel general practitioner surveillance system

This network, part of a more general arrangement for obtaining surveillance information, was initiated in 1984 following a national re-evaluation of communicable disease surveillance (Valleron *et al.* 1986). It was almost certainly the first attempt, within the six countries studied, to use electronic data processing for this purpose on a national scale. Its inception created considerable interest in the global epidemiological community, being described in an *American Journal of Public Health* editorial as 'a new and exciting application of computers in public health'. However, several questions remained unanswered at that time, for example would the enthusiasm for the system decrease over time (Graitcer and Thacker 1986)? In fact, there has been no cause for concern; the number of participating general practitioners has grown from 150 at the commencement of the scheme to 1350 in 2001 (Van Ingen 2001). Newcomers have usually asked to join the network after reading reports of its activities which are regularly published in the medical press (Valleron and Garnerin 1993).

The choice of eight communicable diseases which did not at that time even belong to the list of formally notifiable conditions was clearly a test of the potential effectiveness of this system for motivating the practitioners, although the offer of a free MINITEL to operate the system must have seemed attractive to the initial group who had been selected for this purpose, especially as at that time personal computers were by no means commonplace. Furthermore, those who were designing the development of the system were prepared to take the trouble to consult the doctors to determine their views on how acceptable and practicable such a surveillance network would be, and which diseases they considered important. This support of the surveillance data suppliers, it was considered, was essential if the system were to be successful (Chauvin and Valleron 1995).

Poland

Origins

Any consideration of surveillance must take into account not only the events of the last century but also much earlier events which have had a profound effect on the social, political and economic aspects of life in that country. For example, the first Polish state was established in the tenth century but, after centuries of wars with, and invasions by, neighbouring countries, Poland was eventually partitioned by three occupying powers – Prussia, Russia and Austria – and did not re-emerge as an independent nation until 1918 (Compton 1996). The year 1918, therefore, represents a useful starting point for these considerations for the following reasons.

1 The country was ravaged at that time by epidemics of dysentery, diphtheria, typhoid fever, sexually-transmitted diseases and, above all, *typhus fever*.
2 The first coordinated efforts to control these diseases were made by the creation in 1919 of the Central Epidemiological Institute, an establishment which contained the country's first national diagnostic bacteriological laboratory (Balińska 1998).

In 1923 the Institute was renamed the National Institute of Hygiene (Państwowy Zakład Higieny, usually referred to as PZH), a title which it still holds. As by this time cholera and tuberculosis had been added to the epidemics which the country was experiencing, the main statutory functions assigned to PZH were:

● the diagnosis of infectious diseases
● research on their nature
● reasons for spreading
● methods of control
● the production and experimental studies of sera, vaccines, vaccinia and other bacterial products (Tylewska-Wierzbanowska and Gałązka 1998).

The system of surveillance of epidemics which was introduced by PZH rapidly drew favourable responses from the international community which led to its Director, Ludwik Rajchman, being invited to set up the Health Organization of the League of Nations, of which today's World Health Organization is the direct descendant (Dubin 1995). Increasing needs of the public health service, a wide preventive activity in the control of infectious diseases, control of water and food hygiene, and the necessity of resolving other public health problems in the country were the reasons for establishing 13 branches of PZH in the larger cities and towns. Furthermore, between the two World Wars, PZH had intensified its educational activities by creating, with the assistance of the Rockefeller Foundation, the National School of Hygiene in 1922, the first school of hygiene in Europe. By 1939, 2455 physicians and around 6000 mid-level personnel had been trained there for employment in the public health services.

The Second World War and its aftermath

During the Second World War the German occupation authorities, fearing a spread of infectious diseases, permitted limited and strictly controlled anti-epidemic and other health protection measures (Tylewska-Wierzbanowska and Gałązka 1998). Under communist rule after the War, a Ministry of Health was created in 1945 and healthcare was declared a public responsibility. Administration of the system was strongly centralised but, although the arrangements had many aspects of the Soviet model, private medical practice was never *formally* abolished. Much later, in the 1980s, health sector reforms were linked to efforts to decentralise public services. In the early 1990s (following the major political reforms) these were taken further by the devolution of most public health facilities to the level of each province – the województwo – of which there were 49 and, in the latter part of the decade, even further to each powiat – the traditional district level of local government. From 1 January 1999, new arrangements linked to the establishment of health insurance funds came into being, the main change (from the point of view of this study) being the reduction in the number of województwos from 49 to 16 so that each covered the territory of, on average, about 20 powiats. Therefore the public health infrastructure for communicable disease surveillance has, since then, consisted of PZH, 16 'provincial' health/ epidemiological stations – one per województwo – and 327 'district' units of this kind at powiat level. Notifications of reportable infectious diseases are made by the attending clinician (general practitioner or hospital physician) to the medical director

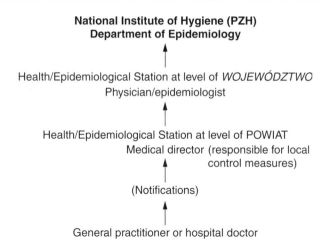

Figure 3.8 Communicable disease surveillance in Poland.

of the powiat health/epidemiological station, a physician with special training and qualifications in epidemiology, who is responsible, along with environmental health officers, for local control measures. Relevant data are then passed to the physician/epidemiologist at the województwo for surveillance purposes and the latter transmits the information to PZH for overall surveillance and monitoring (Magdzik 2000a) (Figure 3.8).

PZH, along with its school of public health, therefore represents a useful combination of a central institution for epidemiological surveillance, public health-oriented medical research and specialised training, assisted by a network of regional, subsidiary outlets (Balińska 2001). For surveillance purposes, the list of notifiable diseases is similar to that in England except that brucellosis, HIV/AIDS, influenza, Legionnaires' disease, Lyme disease, Q fever and trichinellosis are included.

The significance of Poland's location

The choice of Poland for this study perhaps allows more scope for interesting observation than would ordinarily be the case with regard to a single European country. This is at least partly because of its geographical position, having been described over 100 years ago as 'a hyphen between East and West' (Monin 1888) and therefore perceived as the most easterly country in Western Europe (and vice versa). In the West this has traditionally created a perception that most communicable diseases have arrived from the East, in practice through Poland. It is a fact that historically, apart from HIV/AIDS (and possibly poliomyelitis), most of these infections *have* arisen in the East and spread westwards, for example plague, cholera, influenza and typhus (Bourdelais and Dodin 1987). Even in the 1990s, although for a quite specific reason – the release of political prisoners from former Soviet jails – multidrug-resistant tuberculosis can be added to this list. Because of this, in the popular western mind, rightly or wrongly, Eastern Europe has for some time conjured up visions of backwardness and lack of sanitation, a kind of 'breeding-ground' for epidemics (Weindling 2000). However, Poland could be said to have (in the management jargon of the 1960s and 1970s) 'made an opportunity out of a problem' by establishing in 1919, as mentioned earlier, the first national communicable disease surveillance centre in Europe.

Certainly by 1919 there was a need for some country in Central/ Eastern Europe to take the initiative in attempting to make an impact on the typhus epidemic which had begun in Serbia in 1914, but which really took off in 1918/1919 in the wake of the unprecedented migrations which followed the breakdown of law and order in revolutionary Russia. Rather bizarrely, the fact that typhus was coming from communist Russia made for an inextricable link between the notions of 'typhus' and 'bolshevism' which such contrasting figures as Lenin and Churchill both recognised publicly, with Poland being seen as fulfilling a role of *cordon sanitaire* against both infection and communism (Balińska 1995)!

At the end of the Second World War, and of the German occupation, Poland faced multiple problems which were aggravated by great movements of people due to changes of frontiers. Typhus, once more, was the principal communicable disease to cause concern, with an incidence of 66 per 100 000 population in 1945. However, the national surveillance functions of PZH from its temporary base in Łódź (the Warsaw headquarters having been badly damaged during the war) were immediately brought to bear on the situation with the result that, by systematic delousing, within two years the incidence had been reduced to 2 per 100 000 (Kostrzewski and Tylewska-Wierzbanowska 2001).

Diphtheria also represented a major post-war problem, rising in incidence to a peak of 163 per 100 000 population with just under 2000 deaths in 1954, but reduced by painstaking surveillance to a tenth of that incidence within seven years (Gałązka 2001). In the 1990s, and especially after 1992, the country witnessed a problem of re-emerging infections, including diphtheria, transmitted from neighbouring countries to the East, but thereafter the incidence decreased and there has been no evidence of the disease since nine cases in 1996. Currently Poland benefits, in terms of diphtheria surveillance, from being included in a European Laboratory Network organised by the WHO Regional Office for Europe, coordinated by the Central Public Health Laboratory in Colindale (Boriello 2000).

Hepatitis B also deserves a special mention, diagnosed cases having peaked in 1980 at 45 per 100 000 population. However, in 1993 Poland had still the highest incidence (34 per 100 000) of 20 European countries surveyed, but this may have been due in part to the comparatively high level of serological identification, notification and registration of the infection. Unsafe injections in both healthcare settings and drug misuse were considered a major mode of transmission of the virus. The approach to the control of this disease and its success are dealt with later in this book.

Malta

Origins

Cassar (1964) describes how, from the beginning of the nineteenth century, there was a gradual acknowledgement that a number of environmental factors affecting health could best be tackled by a specialised group of doctors. This was put into effect by giving such a group the relevant authority and calling them the 'medical police'. Towards the end of the century the Public Health Department was formed out of this group, the Chief Police Physician becoming the Chief Government Medical Officer; this latter title has remained up to the present day. The disease currently known as brucellosis has some relevance to the origins of surveillance in Malta; indeed one of the illness's previous names was Malta fever. It probably existed there as far back as the sixteenth century, when it was known as 'erratic fever'. As Cassar points out, it was only after the Crimean War ended that the disease assumed significant proportions and, at that time referred to as 'Mediterranean Fever', it was responsible for a great deal of disability among British troops garrisoned there. In 1886 the responsible microbe was identified by Surgeon Major (later Sir) David Bruce at the Station Hospital in Valletta, although it was not until 1905 that it was discovered that the local goats represented the source of infection and that pasteurisation rendered goats' milk safe. British troops were issued with tins of condensed milk because of military doubts concerning the effectiveness of pasteurisation (Cassar 1964). An unexpected disadvantage of this arrangement was an increased incidence of gastrointestinal illness in local young children. Flies 'fresh' from the open sewers would alight on the congealed traces of condensed milk by the holes in the top of the open tins; subsequently young children would touch the same sweet residues and then suck their fingers (Loudon 1998)!

The return of brucellosis

Brucellosis appeared to wish to haunt Malta, as in 1995/1996 the Republic was affected by a major outbreak affecting 240 persons with one death. The infection was transmitted by consumption of ġbejniet (a local delicacy consisting of a small ball of cheese made from unpasteurised milk from sheep or goats and sometimes covered with grains of black pepper). The surveillance of food-borne diseases has been of particular concern in Malta as, not only does the resident population have to be considered, there is also the fact that, for example, during the decade 1985/1995 gross income from tourism trebled (*Malta Information* 1995). However, even before this, increased awareness of the importance of food hygiene and of the need to recognise episodes of preventable food-borne illness were the key reasons for the development of the Food, Drugs and Drinking Water Act of 1972. In 1984/1985, HIV/AIDS appeared first in local residents with coagulation disorders who had received contaminated imported blood products. In March 1986, AIDS became notifiable under the Prevention of Disease Ordinance (1908 as amended) and a National Advisory Committee on AIDS was formed. This led to screening for anti-HIV antibodies in blood and organ donations, tighter criteria for voluntary donation and a drive for the country to become self-sufficient in meeting demands for coagulation factors (Falzon 1998a).

As a consequence of the ongoing reform of the Civil Service which gathered momentum in the early 1990s, the Disease Surveillance Branch was created in 1993 within the new Department of Public Health to deal specifically with notified infectious conditions, and a Principal Medical Officer post was created to head up these activities. In the following year the Department's master plan (Health Vision 2000) was compiled, including targets for infectious disease surveillance which were complementary to the relevant WHO objectives. Following the declaration in 1993 by WHO that tuberculosis represented a global emergency, the Department revised its strategies for screening of persons at increased risk due to occupation, schooling or foreign residence.

In 1994, a number of outbreaks worldwide raised questions concerning the current and future role of the port health services. Re-emergence of plague and cholera in India, diphtheria in the Newly Independent States of the former Soviet Union and the Ebola epidemic in Africa led to, *inter alia*, increased surveillance of incoming passengers and contingency plans were made for the eventuality of importation of viral haemorrhagic fevers or plague into the country; these plans included refurbishment of the 12-bedded infectious ward in one of the state hospitals (Falzon 1998b). It seemed appropriate also, at this time, to have the port health services reviewed in order to find out how best to develop these services and to consider what legislative changes might need to be made. The recommendations following this review covered a range of issues concerning Port Health Regulations, staff training, sampling procedures, etc. but also advised that there should be further development of communicable disease surveillance *throughout the Islands* for the important reason that it had now become difficult to detect most imported infections at the ports (Galbraith 1996). A brief review of the wider existing arrangements for surveillance was carried out later that year (Pollock 1996).

As part of the ongoing development of surveillance, the Department certainly benefited from the global dissemination of new epidemiological software, especially the WHO/CDC Epi-Info series which had been available as 'shareware' for a number of years. This allowed, for example, all the annual figures for notified infectious diseases in Malta from the beginning of the twentieth century to be databased in Windows-readable format, thus simplifying access of data, comparative and time-trend analysis, and generation of reports (Falzon 1998a). Reference was made in Chapter 2 to the fact that, no matter how technologically sophisticated an electronic surveillance system is, its success is largely dependent on the willingness of clinicians to regard notification as a high priority activity on their part. This philosophy has been recognised and accepted in Malta and from the mid-1990s there have been discussions with general practitioners on the possibility of establishing local 'sentinel' surveillance by creating an electronic transmission link between the Disease Surveillance Branch and a number of carefully selected doctors initially, rather as happened in France. The intention is that, eventually, all general practitioners should be able to notify cases by e-mail, and only the priority which the Disease Surveillance Branch is at present having to give to communicable disease issues within the European Union, its networks and working groups, has temporarily delayed progress on this front. (Even though Malta is not at the moment a member of the Union, the Disease Surveillance Branch collaborates with surveillance networks concerned with *Legionella* infections, HIV/AIDS, tuberculosis and meningococcal infections.)

Currently, the list of notifiable infectious diseases closely resembles that of England except that AIDS, brucellosis, *Legionella* infection and Leishmaniasis are additional. Notification is mandatory by law and applies to all doctors in both public and private sectors (Muscat 2001). Malta has three Medical Officers of Health, the British title having been retained even when discarded in the UK, covering, respectively, the South East of the main island (including the port and airport), the North West (containing the main concentration of hotels, restaurants, bars and snackbars) and the separate island of Gozo (essentially a holiday resort). However, all three work from the same central office in the Department of Public Health in Valletta, coordinated by the Principal Medical Officer who is responsible for disease surveillance in the Maltese Islands (Figure 3.9).

Malta is, of course, fortunate in being able to arrange comprehensive surveillance as it has a 'compact' medical community, one main state general hospital and one medical school, along with a flourishing weekly professional/social get-together under the auspices of the Medical Association of Malta.

**Principal Medical Officer (Disease Surveillance), Department of Public Health
Three Medical Officers of Health**

Notifications

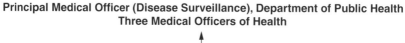

Clinicians in South East and North West Malta, and Island of Gozo

Figure 3.9 Communicable disease surveillance in Malta.

Uganda

Origins

Organised national communicable disease surveillance in Uganda is of comparatively recent origin, as is described below. Any study of the development of surveillance must take into account a situation which is, on the face of it, rather paradoxical. The country is still struggling to recover from decades of civil strife of a most brutal kind and yet there is now political and social stability, along with considerable evidence of a vigorous programme of redevelopment, in which public health features prominently and in which maximum delegation of responsibility to district level or below is a marked element (Lwamafa 2002a). Iliffe (1998) describes how Idi Amin's military tyranny which was established in 1971 had a devastating effect not only on the state and the economy, but also on the medical profession itself and the medical school at Makerere University in Kampala, which had generally flourished during the first decade of independence. Even when the military regime was overthrown in 1979, peace and recovery were still far away and the need for rehabilitation of the nation's health services was great. It is salutary to consider that priority had to be given to restoring such basic services as water, plumbing and sewerage, although United Nations International Children's Emergency Fund (UNICEF) provided funds for elementary refurbishment of around 100 health centres. Even when in 1984, as Iliffe points out, a very observant district medical officer in Rakai District along with physicians at the Mulago teaching hospital were comparing a clinical condition known locally as 'Slim' with the syndrome of AIDS as seen in the United States, Uganda was in the midst of civil war and relevant news items did not reach the Press until the Government of former President of Uganda, Milton Obote, was overthrown in September 1985.

Against this background it is remarkable to observe that, in spite of the devastation of the past, the Ministry of Health has been able to commit itself to a 5-year Health Sector Strategic Plan (2000/01–2004/05). This, for the purposes of this study, includes active programmes on the prevention and control of communicable diseases, especially malaria, HIV/AIDS and tuberculosis which are among the most common causes of illness and death across Uganda's age profile (Ministry of Health, Uganda 1995).

Nevertheless, the reality is that Uganda is still one of the least developed countries; 44% of the population live below the poverty line and, to quote from the Strategic Plan, 'geographical access to healthcare facilities is so far limited to only 49% of households'. Similarly, a Health Inventory carried out in 2000 showed that only 42.7% of parishes in the country had any form of health facility. Understandably, microbiological laboratory facilities are limited, except in association with certain Government District Hospitals.

Developments since 1995

Organised national communicable disease surveillance in its present form really only began around the year 1995, although it has continued to evolve and improve ever since. An assessment of the surveillance systems in the country took place in 2000 and was soon followed by the 5-year plan of action to address the gaps revealed by the assessment. Being considerably influenced by the above factors, the surveillance systems demonstrate their own unique approach. The philosophy accepted by all concerned is that 'effective communicable disease control relies on effective surveillance which is necessary to monitor diseases with a high burden, to detect outbreaks of epidemic-prone nature and to monitor progress towards national or international control/eradication targets' (Epidemiological Surveillance Division 2001).

To support these functions, case definitions and action thresholds have been developed and updated, taking into account advice from CDC Atlanta and WHO Geneva, to help health workers and others at all levels to detect and report the country's priority diseases for appropriate and timely action. The case definitions have been very thoughtfully devised, making a distinction between:

- those composed to assist local communities in bringing suspicious illness to the attention of a health facility, and
- those developed for use *at the health facility itself* as thresholds for action.

For example, in the former list, the case definition of measles is simply 'any person with fever and rash', whereas in the latter it is 'generalised maculopapular skin rash and fever of at least 38°C and at least one of the following: red eyes (conjunctivitis), red lips and sore mouth (stomatitis) or cough and runny nose (coryza)'. Similarly, the *community* case definition of AIDS is simply 'a chronic disease characterised by fever, weight loss and diarrhoea', whereas the *health facility* version is 'either disseminated Kaposi's sarcoma or cryptococcal meningitis, or two major symptoms (weight loss, diarrhoea or fever for more than one month) plus one minor symptom/sign (e.g. oral thrush, herpes zoster, generalised lymph node enlargement)' (ESD 2001).

It is important to realise that at the present time, while microbiological facilities below district level are not well developed, these surveillance case definitions form the basis of most notifications; this situation is likely to continue for some time, until the capacity for laboratory confirmation can be strengthened (Lamunu 2002). Accordingly communicable diseases of public health importance tend to be reported in the following manner.

Residents of a village may be the first to notice an unusually high number of cases in a locality. In these circumstances the hope is that the matter will be reported to a 'community resource person', such as a teacher or religious leader who, in turn, is expected to pass on the information to the person in charge of the nearest peripheral health facility, for example the parish nurse, for initial investigation. If the episode settles down, the matter will probably receive no further consideration. However, if the nurse is concerned, the opinion of the nearest clinical officer (medical assistant) at sub-county level can be obtained. If that individual, in turn, considers that the outbreak is one of real significance, for example has epidemic potential or appears to be one of the diseases targeted for eradication or elimination, such as acute flaccid paralysis/poliomyelitis, an urgent report (notification) by telephone, 'walkie-talkie' or by hand is made within 24 hours to the doctor based at county level, where there may also be a laboratory technician. If the relevant threshold for notification is reached, a similar immediate report is also sent by the county to the Epidemiological Surveillance Division (ESD) of the Ministry of Health in Kampala. The ESD is responsible for national communicable disease surveillance within the overall programme of the National Disease Control Department. However, if the ESD considers that the outbreak is likely to have wider than local distribution, or that in some other way it has major significance (e.g. an outbreak of cholera), one of the Division's epidemiologists will visit the area to assist with the investigation and the implementation of the public health intervention.

The county level is one of considerable operational importance as this is the first level at which a doctor is available and not only does this person attend the various health centres as a clinician,

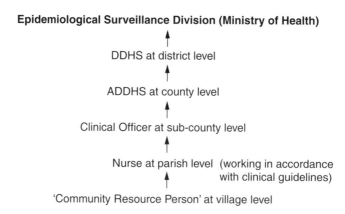

Figure 3.10 Communicable disease surveillance in Uganda.

the role also includes the responsibility, as Assistant District Director of Health Services (ADDHS), for all necessary measures to control local outbreaks. The latter represents a comparatively recent delegation of responsibility from the District Director of Health Services (DDHS). Previously the district itself represented the lowest level to which the control function had been delegated. The other reason for the county level's importance is that it represents the local Parliamentary Constituency, with one or two Members of Parliament who, understandably, tend to take a considerable interest in local outbreaks affecting their voters.

The district, with an average population of around 500 000, represents the level of local government and each has a government hospital with an average of 100 beds, a medical superintendent in charge and most having laboratory facilities. The district's public health service is headed by a DDHS, appointed by the District Service Commission, who has received appropriate postgraduate training leading to for example the Master of Public Health (MPH) degree. The operational relationship in public health matters between the district and the county is a flexible one which allows the DDHS and ADDHS to work as a team but the official reporting channel to the ESD is through the DDHS (Figure 3.10). Reporting/notification of surveillance data to the ESD takes place within three time-scales.

1 *Immediate notification* (within 24 hours) by telephone, by radio-call or by fax, if the condition is an 'eradicable disease' or has epidemic potential.
2 *Weekly compilation*: sent by radio call (70%), by telephone (25%) or by fax (5%).

3 *Monthly reporting* of all infectious diseases seen in the relevant health facility during the month.

The above systems constitute the main source and flow of surveillance data but they do not, of course, preclude notification by a general medical practitioner, hospital doctor or laboratory microbiologist. The surveillance database used at the ESD is Epi-Info Version 6 but conversion to Epi-Info 2000 is imminent.

The value of relevant feedback is fully appreciated by the ESD and this is provided on a weekly basis to districts on the understanding that they, in turn, will pass the information 'down the line'. The ESD also purchases space each Monday in the authoritative daily newspaper *New Vision* so that, among other things, the public can be made aware of the incidence of communicable diseases in each district. Consolidated information is made available in a quarterly publication by the ESD itself.

The ESD does not exist in isolation within the Ministry of Health. It lies within the National Disease Control Department which, in turn, is one of five Departments of the Clinical Services and Community Health Directorate, one of two Directorates, the other being concerned with planning, development and quality assurance. The ESD's closest and most important links are, via the National Disease Control Department, with the Community Health Department as both have certain overlapping responsibilities in the general field of communicable disease epidemiology, response and control of outbreaks, in addition to health education and immunisation.

European/WHO collaboration in surveillance

A comparatively recent development is the establishment of a number of international collaborations in surveillance. The development of the European Community, an area with mobility of labour and increasing travel, has increased the possibility of outbreaks of communicable disease which transcend national boundaries. Although this study focuses mainly on the evolution of surveillance systems in six individual countries, each with its own 'culture', one cannot ignore the very considerable benefits that have accrued from international networking. Although *informal* professional cooperation was well established by the early 1990s, in September 1998 a decision of the European Parliament and of the Council established collaboration on a formal basis. This directive acknowledged that the surveillance, prevention and control of communicable diseases was to represent a priority for community action and invited the commission to set up a trans-frontier network (to be known as the European Network for Epidemiological Surveillance and Control of Communicable Diseases) to devise working definitions of notifiable diseases, to collect, update, analyse and disseminate member states' data on such diseases and to work with national and international agencies (particularly WHO) on these matters. However, in accordance with the principle of subsidiarity, such measures were to be taken by the community only if the objectives could be better achieved by it than by the member states themselves. The network at community level was to be used for epidemiological surveillance of the relevant diseases and an early warning and response system for their prevention and control. Member states were to consult one another, in liaison with the commission, with a view to coordinating their efforts for the prevention and control of communicable diseases. The costs resulting from the operation of the network at community level were to be met from community resources, although costs arising from the operation of the network at national level were to be financed by the member states themselves.

Network-related projects on disease-specific surveillance are listed below.

List 1
EWGLI (legionellosis)
Enter-Net (salmonellosis, and infection with *E. coli* 0157)
Euro TB (tuberculosis)
EuroHIV (HIV/AIDS)
EISS (influenza)
ENIVD (imported viral haemorrhagic fevers)
EARSS (antimicrobial resistance)
Helics (nosocomial infections)

List 2
Hepatitis C
Campylobacteriosis
European bacterial meningitis surveillance system
EUVAC-NET (measles, pertussis, infection with *H. influenzae*)
Zoonoses (brucellosis, rabies)

CHAPTER 4

Prevention

When one moves from the sphere of surveillance to that of prevention, in comparing different countries one begins to detect not only a measure of social concern which is wider than that of professionals alone but also different cultural environments which can have a bearing on both legal requirements and realms of personal choice. As mentioned in Chapter 2, the term 'prevention', in this book, relates essentially to measures taken to protect susceptible individuals and therefore relates mainly, but not exclusively, to immunisation procedures.

Immunisation

These procedures are aimed at reducing morbidity and mortality from vaccine-preventable diseases. Although immunisation procedures may be offered to the whole of a population or to special target groups, such as young children, personnel in certain high risk occupations, military recruits, travellers or refugees, this study focuses on routine childhood immunisation as, perhaps, the best means of illustrating the cultural differences referred to. The most striking example of the latter is the fact that of the six countries examined only England and Uganda have totally informal, voluntary arrangements, the other four depending on legal requirements, or other obligations, for some or all of these procedures; one perhaps unforeseen consequence of the English approach is described later in this chapter. As the range of diseases which are actually or potentially vaccine-preventable is quite large, this account will focus, *for comparative purposes*, on a limited number although the actual schedules may vary from country to country, including all or most of the following:

- diphtheria
- pertussis

- tetanus
- poliomyelitis
- measles
- mumps
- rubella
- *Haemophilus influenzae* type b
- tuberculosis
- hepatitis B.

It should not be forgotten that, in addition to protecting the individual from developing a serious disease, immunisation procedures also help to protect the community by reducing the spread of infectious agents and, if sufficiently widely applied, may provide indirect protection to some *non*-immunised persons within the community by the development of herd immunity. This aspect is explored to some extent in Chapter 6. In recent years a clearer understanding of the extent to which herd immunity can be created has been derived from applications of mathematical modelling which have also been useful in designing cost-effective strategies for the prevention of these diseases. Computing such factors as the probability of infection on contact, the rate of contact and the duration of infectivity can help to predict epidemic behaviour, and also to offer guidance on for example the optimum age for beginning a course of immunisation and the ideal gaps between procedures.

England

The attitude to immunisation in England is almost certain to have been significantly influenced by the particular history of smallpox vaccination: its origin; the attempts of the Government to encourage it, leading in due course to compulsory vaccination; the development of the anti-vaccination lobby; and the eventual withdrawal of compulsion as recently as 1948 – with the implementation of the NHS Act 1946, i.e. seven years after the introduction nationally of the first element of the modern childhood immunisation schedule, the diphtheria antigen. It is perhaps worth looking at this historical factor in a little detail.

Throughout the nineteenth century, smallpox vaccination caused considerable controversy in England. The Government's support for the procedure had led to the Vaccination Acts of 1840, 1841 and 1853 making vaccination successively universal, free and finally compulsory for all children within the first year of life.

However, public disquiet was widespread and a Bill of 1866, aimed at consolidating the statutes for compulsion, was withdrawn as 'the measure was likely to meet with great opposition and it was very doubtful whether it could be carried through Parliament' (Stern 1927). Further legislative action was undertaken five years later when the disease had once more assumed epidemic proportions but subsequent public demonstrations against compulsion, including riots in Leicester, rendered the law relatively ineffective. The introduction of a concept of 'conscientious objection', which had to be supported by a sworn declaration before a Justice of the Peace, represented a compromise which appeared generally acceptable. Interestingly, in 1948 when all legislation with regard to compulsion was withdrawn, *this was only implicit* as, quite simply, there was no reference to compulsion in the 1946 Act. However, there may well be a further factor of a cultural nature operating which could be influencing the English attitude; this is outlined in Chapter 6.

Thus routine childhood immunisation in England, in contrast to many other countries including, for the purposes of this study, the United States, France, Malta and Poland, has in recent years been totally free from compulsion, direct or indirect, and is secured informally by education, information-giving, persuasion and good organisation within primary healthcare (including, more recently, financial incentives for general practitioners to achieve specific targets). Clearly, then, in England vigorous health promotion activities are essential to increase public knowledge of both the relevant diseases and the protective vaccines, to promote a positive attitude to immunisation; similar considerations apply to Uganda, as is shown later.

Protection against diphtheria, the first element of the twentieth century routine childhood immunisation programme, was in fact not introduced very early. Although in July 1922 the Ministry of Health had issued a memorandum on the supply and administration of diphtheria antitoxin, with a follow-up memorandum 10 years later, only a small number of MOHs introduced the procedure into their maternity and child welfare centres. This delay in introducing a valuable preventive measure was largely due to the absorption of MOHs in day-to-day matters of hospital administration and also to their reluctance to try to persuade local councils to incur additional expenditure in the financially straitened circumstances of the 1930s (Lewis 1991). However, with the onset of the Second World War the Ministry of Health introduced its *Memorandum on the Production of Artificial Immunity against Diphtheria*

(Ministry of Health 1940) and by the end of that year undertook free provision of the antigen, thereby ending any burden on the local rates.

The national immunisation scheme was finally implemented in 1941; deaths from diphtheria fell by one third within a year and incidence and mortality were down by three quarters by 1946 (Holland and Stewart 1997). By the end of the war the Ministry had issued 30 circulars on the subject. In conjunction with the Ministry of Information, it was responsible for a series of posters, radio talks and advertisements in both national and local newspapers, for the purpose of encouraging parents to have their children immunised. By the end of 1944, as was revealed in the report of the Chief Medical Officer of the Ministry of Health for the years 1939–1945, 2 069 377 children under the age of five years, and 3 296 578 between the ages of five and 15 had had the procedure (Ministry of Health 1946). On 5 July 1948, with the coming into being of the NHS, immunisation became a function of the local health authorities and the benefit of this was evident in the improved take-up in 1949 in comparison with the previous year (Ministry of Health 1951). However, it is important to realise that delaying the national scheme until 1941, although evidence of the effectiveness of the procedure was available in 1930, could be considered to have resulted in some 20 000 avoidable deaths from the disease during that decade (Holland and Stewart 1997). Nevertheless by 2001/2002, 94% of children had been immunised against diphtheria (and also tetanus and poliomyelitis, as these three procedures are normally carried out at the same time) by their second birthday (Department of Health 2002).

It is perhaps appropriate at this point to draw attention to the fact that the reasons for the decline in mortality from infectious diseases have been the subject of fierce debate. In particular, Professor Thomas McKeown of Birmingham University demonstrated in 1976 that improvements in the standard of living, especially in nutrition, which raised the potential victim's resistance to air-borne diseases, were reducing mortality from such conditions before the advent of immunisation and chemotherapy (Lewis 1991). He argued that, with the exception of vaccination against smallpox, immunisation had *not* been the most important influence on mortality, pointing instead to improvements in nutrition and hygiene. However, he concluded that although mortality was already in decline, the fall became more rapid as new vaccines were introduced (McKeown 1979).

Vaccines against whooping cough, made from whole, killed *B.*

pertussis, were developed before the Second World War and large-scale clinical trials in the late 1940s and 1950s (Allwright 1988) demonstrated the safety and potency of three doses of certain of these products. Prior to the availability of pertussis immunisation in the 1950s, the average annual number of notifications of the disease in England and Wales exceeded 100 000. However, less than two decades later when vaccine coverage was over 80%, there were only 2069 notifications in 1972. Within three years coverage rates had fallen to 30% as a result of public anxiety about the safety of the vaccine, and major epidemics, with over 100 000 notified cases, followed in 1977/79 and 1981/83 (DoH 1996). The National Childhood Encephalopathy Study was set up to investigate the possibility of neurological damage from the vaccine and in the wake of the report of the Royal Commission on Civil Liability and Compensation for Personal Injury the Government decided that there should be a scheme of payments for vaccine damage. The subsequent return of professional and public confidence led to increased take-up of the vaccine, cutting short the next epidemic which died away in 1986, well below the levels of the previous two. By 2001/2002, 93% of children had been immunised by their second birthday (Department of Health 2002).

Until the introduction of the measles vaccine in 1968 annual notifications varied between 160 000 and 800 000, the peaks occurring predictably in two-year cycles. However, take-up of the vaccine was never sufficiently high to have an effect on virus transmission and by the late 1980s annual notifications had fallen only to between 50 000 and 100 000 (DoH 1996). In countries such as the USA, where high coverage was achieved quite early, very low levels of measles were observed, a situation which did not pass without comment in England. The District Medical Officer for the City of Coventry (the author) ran a poster campaign during 1985 with the message:

'**Question**: What can you get in Coventry that you can't get in New York, San Francisco or Los Angeles?
Answer: MEASLES!'

Also, along with two colleagues, he had a letter published in the *Lancet* with the title 'Measles – there ought to be a law against it!' (Middleton *et al.* 1985). It was only following the introduction of the combined measles/mumps/rubella (MMR) vaccine in 1988, with its particular appeal, at that time, to parents (because of one antigen protecting against three diseases; in practice two injections instead of six) that coverage levels in excess of 90% were soon achieved.

A possible link between the MMR immunisation and autism was suggested by a group of researchers at the Royal Free Hospital in London (Wakefield *et al.* 1998). However, in spite of the fact that extensive independent studies carried out subsequently – most recently a very carefully undertaken Danish study involving more than half a million children (Madsen *et al.* 2002) – have shown that there is no association between autism and MMR vaccination, the continuing adverse publicity in the media concerning the alleged effects of the procedure has resulted in decreased public confidence in the safety of the vaccine. This has led to a coverage of only 87% in 2000/2001 and 84% in 2001/2002, i.e. 8% lower than the peak coverage of 92% achieved in 1995/1996 (Department of Health 2002). Slight falls in coverage of diphtheria, tetanus, poliomyelitis, pertussis and *Haemophilus influenzae* protection were also observed during this period, probably as a result of a 'halo effect' operating in reverse. This situation illustrates what a recent editorial in the *BMJ* has referred to as 'the discomfort of patient power' in which patients may choose to disregard their doctors' advice and do something that their doctors regard as odd, even crazy. The editorial concludes that doctors will have to live with 'irrational' decisions by the public (Smith 2002).

A comment by Dr Wakefield, at the press conference to launch his controversial 1998 paper, to the effect that single vaccines might be safer (although he put forward no evidence to support this theory) has led some parents to demand that this approach be adopted. The Department of Health has rejected this idea on the grounds that the general body of medical advice, including that of WHO, is that MMR is both safe and effective, and the time lapse between three separate injections would leave more children exposed to infection. Although these points form the basis of the Department of Health's message, there is some anecdotal evidence that, paradoxically, the more insistent the reassurance the more some persons distrust the advice, perhaps partly because they find it difficult to draw the line between Government and medical professionals' advice. A few general practitioners have offered single antigens, *on a private basis* as such an arrangement does not constitute any part of NHS provision, but this is considered an undesirable professional practice.

Before the introduction of immunisation against *Haemophilus influenzae* infections, these were an important cause of morbidity and mortality especially in young children; one in every 600 children developing some form of invasive disease before their fifth birthday. Since the introduction of immunisation, disease incidence has fallen dramatically (DoH 1996). By 2001/2002, 93% of children had been immunised by their second birthday (Department of Health 2000).

The Joint Committee on Vaccination and Immunisation advises the Department of Health on immunisation policy and full details of schedules are published in the latter's publication *Immunisation against Infectious Disease*. The country ratified the fifth objective of the *Health For All in the year 2000* programme of WHO Europe which states: 'By the year 2000, there should be no indigenous cases of poliomyelitis, diphtheria, neonatal tetanus, measles, mumps and congenital rubella in the Region'. Clearly the recent decrease in the take-up of MMR vaccine is getting in the way of further progress with regard to these diseases.

Key features of the arrangements in England are that immunisation is free of charge within the NHS and that virtually all the procedures are carried out by the child's general practitioner. (On a day-to-day basis, it is frequently carried out by a practice nurse, but with the doctor retaining overall clinical responsibility.) For example, in Coventry the figure is 100% (Bardhan 1999) and in Birmingham the only immunisation procedures *not* undertaken by a general practitioner are for the small number of children whose parents have not registered with one (Blair 1999). When a child's birth is reported, a duplicate notification alerts the PCT Child Health System, which in turn allocates the child to a general practitioner, usually the same one as that providing primary care for the mother. This process enrols the child in the Child Health System's computerised database that schedules the immunisations, calculates local coverage and identifies defaulters. By the time a newborn child is 10 days old the parents will have been visited by a Health Visitor who discusses the immunisation arrangements and seeks their consent for the child to be entered into a computer-based programme, thereby satisfying data protection requirements (Salisbury 1999). Until the 1980s, only about 50% of children were immunised in general practitioner surgeries; the remainder had the procedures carried out in child health clinics of the local health authority.

[The transition to 100% general practice was not necessarily achieved smoothly or easily. While the author was District Medical Officer of Coventry, he had to argue the case quite strongly with some members of the local Community Health Council who felt that they were being deprived of a valued facility, as clinic times were often more convenient than general practitioner surgery hours. Nevertheless he was able, eventually, to convince them of the overriding benefits of having the procedures carried out by the doctor who would be familiar with all relevant aspects of the family medical history and who would moreover be the one called out if the child were to develop any acute reaction which might worry the parents.]

A 1987 Government White Paper, *Promoting Better Health*, has probably had a significant role in continuing to improve immunisation coverage in that it led to the introduction of new general practitioner contracts which included targets for immunisation of children on their practice lists, the achievement of which had relevance to part of the practice's remuneration. For example, the maximum remuneration for this sector of work is received only if the coverage is at least 90%, and if it is less than 70% no specific remuneration is forthcoming. Paradoxically, there have been a few public expressions of concern in the national Press at this method of remuneration, as far as MMR immunisation is concerned, to the effect that 'doctors are being bribed to carry out the Government's policy!'.

Figure 2.3 (*see* p 21) offers one illustration of the interaction between preventive and surveillance activities. Evaluation of the immunisation service is extremely important to assess coverage, the incidence of vaccine-preventable diseases and public satisfaction with the service. Coverage is evaluated by the COVER method (Cover of Vaccination Evaluated Rapidly). Completed forms giving details of the procedures carried out are returned from the general practitioner's surgery to the Child Health System of the local PCT; this is the system which also receives details of birth notification and generates the invitations for the child's immunisations. Aggregated data are then sent on quarterly to the PHLS Communicable

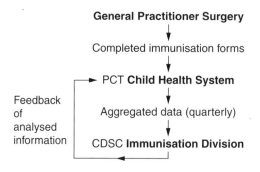

Figure 4.1 Monitoring of immunisation coverage in England.

Disease Surveillance Centre which, on behalf of the Department of Health, publishes the summarised information on a quarterly basis. The main purpose of the COVER scheme is to improve coverage by providing the PCT's District Immunisation Coordinator (usually, but not invariably, the CCDC) with relevant and timely information, but it is also a useful means of detecting local or national changes in coverage (Begg *et al.* 1989) (Figure 4.1).

United States

The involvement of legislation in this field can be noted as far back as the early nineteenth century when Massachusetts passed a law which required the general population to be vaccinated against smallpox. During the next 100 years the procedure became more widely accepted, although opposing voices were also raised in the interests of the rights of individuals. However, the decision of the Supreme Court in 1905, supporting the right of states to legislate in this sector, led in 1922 to a further enactment, specifying that the procedure could be required prior to school entry (Orenstein *et al.* 1991). The special significance of this latter factor is that it has formed the continuing basis for immunisation policy in the United States and routine childhood immunisation on this obligatory basis appears to be generally accepted, as shown later.

Federal support for immunisation has represented a prominent feature, especially since 1955 when inactivated poliovaccine became available. From the Presidency of John F Kennedy onwards, individual presidents have been keen to be publicly associated with specific initiatives to improve immunisation coverage – Kennedy in 1962, Jimmy Carter in 1976, George Bush in 1991 and Bill Clinton in 1993. Occasionally, such initiatives have had declared objectives in terms of coverage, for example 90% of all children by 1979 and 90% of *pre-school* children by 1998. Both of these targets have been achieved. A key feature of the federal arrangements is that 'no child can be denied immunisation because of parental inability to pay any fee' (Orenstein *et al.* 1999). Currently, recommendations regarding immunisation of children are developed by collaboration between the Advisory Committee on Immunization Practices and the American Academies of Pediatrics and Family Physicians. Immunisations are currently provided through both the private (about 2/3) and public sectors (about 1/3).

Using the State of Oklahoma as *illustrative* (as in Chapter 3), the routine childhood immunisation programme represents part of a federal government initiative and is therefore centrally funded excluding, of course, those parents who choose to obtain this service from private physicians. Apart from the latter, immunisation is offered at child health clinics provided locally by the county health departments and also from the specialised facilities serving the Native American population. The basic schedule comprises protection against diphtheria, pertussis, tetanus, poliomyelitis, measles, mumps, rubella (in MMR form), *Haemophilus influenzae* type b and hepatitis B; BCG vaccine is not offered routinely. Evidence of immunisation has to be produced before any child is allowed to enter kindergarten, school or any other child group facility such as a day-care centre, although there are certain exceptions, mentioned below. In the Spring of each year in which the child is due to enter in the Fall, during the 'kindergarten round-up' the immunisation status is checked so that any missing procedures can be carried out. Although the State retains the overall responsibility for the achievement of the programme, the local schools and other centres are the 'enforcing agencies' on the State's behalf. Exemptions are allowed only on the basis of authenticated medical (as in all states), religious (as in some but not all states) or personal grounds (as in only a few states); fewer than 1% of the State's children fall into these categories. [This is in keeping with the findings of a survey of 40 states which showed that persons with any kind of exemption under state law, including medical contraindications, accounted for only an average of 0.64% (Orenstein *et al.* 1999).]

The monthly *Epidemiological Bulletin* produced by the State Department of Health, referred to earlier in Chapter 3, routinely includes the details of the immunisation schedule including information on topics which are frequently the subject of questions from healthcare professionals, school staff and parents: vaccine handling and storage, delays occurring between individual immunisation procedures, requirements for older children, etc. (Pollock 1992). Nationally, low take-up rates tend to be associated with low educational level of parents, low socio-economic status, large family size, young parental age and non-white race or ethnicity (Orenstein 1998). However, to a certain extent, a quite separate arrangement tends to counteract missing out on this protection, namely the federal means-tested food voucher system for needy infants and young children as they have to be examined periodically, including an assessment of immunisation status, as a condition of entitlement.

Although immunisations are undertaken by both private physicians and public sector providers, epidemiological aspects, such as communicable disease surveillance and outbreak control, remain the responsibility of health departments and other public sector agencies. Coverage of immunisation of school entrants is readily obtainable by surveys of schools and day-care centres, given the arrangements described above. With regard to pre-school children, coverage is estimated through the National Immunization Survey. The information is obtained every year by telephone and relates to a random sample of about 33 000 children aged 19–35 months. Actual disease reduction is evaluated by the reporting, by state health departments, of the 10 vaccine-preventable diseases to the National Notifiable Disease Surveillance System (NNDSS) (Orenstein 1998). The following figures from the CDC represent coverage in 2001, by the second birthday.

Diphtheria	94%
Tetanus	94%
Pertussis	94%
Poliomyelitis	89%
Hepatitis B	89%
Hib	93%
MMR	91%
Varicella	76%

France

Two national professional bodies, the Conseil Supérieur d'Hygiène Publique de France and the Comité Technique des Vaccinations, are together responsible for advising the Minister of Health on all matters concerning vaccination policy. A central element of routine childhood immunisation is governed by legislation – la législation vaccinale – by which 'a certain number of immunisations are rendered obligatory by texts of law', in effect, a series of laws incorporated in the Code de la Santé Publique (Ministère de la Santé Publique 1995). This applies to protection against diphtheria (since 1938), tetanus (since 1940), tuberculosis (since 1950) and poliomyelitis (since 1964). This compulsory element stems from a period during which the incidence of these diseases was still significant in France and is currently implemented by having these procedures as a requirement for entry into kindergarten or school (Euvax 2001). The formal requirement to have two other vaccinations, namely against smallpox and typhoid fever, no longer exists because of global eradication of the former disease and improvement of living standards greatly reducing the risk of the latter. However, perhaps one ought to be aware that, with regard to attitudes to immunisation arrangements in France, Michel Rey (1980) has written that these reflect the 'Latin tradition of countries of the South with their Mediterranean culture and legalistic inclination, relying on laws but being sufficiently latitudinarian with regard to their application'. This aspect will be explored a little in Chapter 6.

Certain other procedures while not compulsory come under the heading of 'recommended': vaccination against pertussis, *Haemophilus influenzae* type b, hepatitis B, measles, mumps and rubella. The view is that success in having this latter group of vaccinations carried out should come about as a result of 'health education based on encouraging individual responsibility'. The completion of these procedures is recorded in the child's *Carnet de Santé*, literally 'Health Notebook' (Ministère de l'Emploi et de la Solidarité 1999). As in the case of England, France ratified, on behalf of the European Region of WHO, the fifth objective of *Health For All in the year 2000* but, in addition to the six diseases included in the Declaration, added pertussis, infections by *Haemophilus influenzae* type b, childhood tuberculosis and hepatitis B (Ministère de la Santé Publique 1995).

The majority of routine childhood immunisation procedures are carried out by private medical practitioners, i.e. general practitioners or paediatricians, 85% according to a survey carried out in 1989 (Ministère de la Santé Publique 1995), rising to 90% ten years later (Institut de Veille Sanitaire 1999). The public health sector is involved to a variable extent according to the individual département, through Protection Maternelle et Infantile (PMI) centres, municipal dispensaries and immunisation centres, the immunisations being carried out there as a part of routine 'child protection' consultations (Institut de Veille Sanitaire 2000). The responsibility for seeing that the obligatory immunisation procedures are carried out lies with the Conseil Général of each individual département, a democratically elected body with certain allocated health and social responsibilities (Code général des collectivités 1997). By a decree in 1984, the former included immunisation, except in the case of those communes which had a well established service and wished to retain this (Ecole Nationale de Santé Publique 1995). As was mentioned in Chapter 3, the département is the level at which the Médecin Inspecteur de Santé Publique is employed, and it is therefore convenient to have immunisation responsibility located there; Chapter 5 (on Control) describes how this is also the level at which outbreaks of communicable disease are tackled.

Immunisation coverage is evaluated by the analysis of the health certificates of infants aged 24 months; these have to be completed as part of the obligatory health assessment undertaken at that age. However, as recently as the mid-1990s it was acknowledged that, although exhaustive in theory, in practice only 55–60% of these records could be reliably used for this purpose and a good deal of estimating had to be carried out, for example by recording the number of doses of antigen issued in relation to the numbers of children eligible. Accordingly, the medical profession was at that time being exhorted to adopt a more responsible attitude to this potentially extremely valuable form of record keeping (Guérin 1996). Currently the evaluation of coverage by analysis of PMI data at the level of the département is amplified by scrutiny of research studies commissioned by the Ministry of Health (Institut de Veille Sanitaire 2000). However, the Ministère de la Santé Publique is aware of possible flaws in evaluating coverage and has stated (1999) that, in addition to the above-mentioned problems of the individual records themselves, the latter are also at risk because of the 'qualité du circuit de transmission des certificats' and for these reasons the Ministère itself has stated (1999) 'les chiffres obtenus doivent être interprétés avec précaution' (the figures obtained require to be interpreted with caution).

Against this background the following represent the figures for coverage in 2000, at age 24 months (Ministère de la Santé, 02/08/02).

Diphtheria + Tetanus	98.1%	Compulsory
Poliomyelitis*	98.0%	Compulsory
Tuberculosis (BCG)	83.1%	Compulsory before entry into any child care group or organisation, and in any event before 6 years of age
Pertussis	97.4%	Recommended
Hib	86.1%	Recommended
HBV	26.0%	Recommended
Measles ⎫	84.1%	Recommended
Rubella ⎬ Mostly as MMR	83.8%	Recommended
Mumps ⎭	83.5%	Recommended

* Only *inactivated* poliovaccine is used routinely; live oral vaccine is reserved for epidemic situations.

Malta

A quirk of fate has a bearing on immunisation as far as Malta is concerned. In 1798 Napoleon, with mastery of the Mediterranean as his objective, invaded the Maltese Islands and, displacing the Knights of St John, immediately began to promulgate new laws. Even though he remained there for only six days and the French occupation lasted only two years, some important elements of the Code Napoleon, with their public health implications, rubbed off on to local legislation (Falzon 1998a). Accordingly it is not too surprising to find that routine childhood immunisation against diphtheria, tetanus and poliomyelitis is described in an appropriate Ordinance as the 'duty of the parent or other person having the custody of any child who has attained the relevant age and who has not already been completely protected in accordance with the provisions of this section to the satisfaction of the Superintendent of Public Health, and that failure to comply with this duty will result in the parent being summoned by the Commissioner of Police to appear before the Court of Magistrates of Judicial Police so that, if considered appropriate, the child may be immunised by Order of Court' (Prevention of Disease Ordinance 1908 – as amended). Routine childhood immunisation is offered by the Government's Department of Primary Health Care and is mostly (about 65–70%) undertaken, free of charge, in Government Health Centres, the main one being situated, in association with the Head-quarters of the National Immunisation Service, in Floriana on the outskirts of Valletta, the capital. The remainder choose to have the procedures carried out by general practitioners or paediatricians in private practice. The immunisation status of each child is assessed by the scrutiny of child health records and any omissions are promptly followed up. Coverage is evaluated by examination of child health records at 24 months and these records are considered totally reliable, perhaps a benefit of being a small country with a close-knit medical community. The following represent the 2000 figures, obtained from the National Immunisation Service.

Diphtheria/Tetanus	92.3%
Poliomyelitis	92.1%
Pertussis	91.1%
MMR	85.3%
Hib	91.3%

Poland

Poland has a strong tradition of combatting diseases by vaccination wherever possible. When the National Institute of Hygiene, Państwowy Zakład Higieny (PZH), was created in 1923, out of the Central Epidemiological Institute, its initial statutory functions included '... the production and experimental studies of sera, vaccines, vaccinia and other bacterial products'. Accordingly, a special Department of Sera and Vaccines Production was soon established at PZH, in which, in due course, 32 vaccines were produced including those against cholera, bacillary dysentery (shigellosis), typhoid, smallpox and rabies, along with 10 immune sera including those against diphtheria, tetanus, shigella and streptococci. The League of Nations used PZH's vaccines for its preventive campaigns in Russia and Greece, and during the German occupation in the Second World War the Polish underground, under cover of performing official functions, was able to produce typhus vaccine clandestinely at PZH for the Polish population including prisoners in concentration camps (Tylewska-Wierzbanowska and Gałązka 1998)!

Routine childhood immunisation in Poland – against tuberculosis, diphtheria/tetanus, pertussis, poliomyelitis, measles and hepatitis B – is obligatory and is carried out by general practitioners, free of charge. The only exception to the latter is when the parents want the child to have a procedure which is not included in the schedule, for example *acellular* pertussis vaccine (Korycka 2002a). The word 'obligatory' (obowiązkowe in Polish) implies a duty or obligation. Interestingly enough, it does not mean *compulsory* (przymusowe in Polish) which implies compulsion *by force if necessary*, a concept unacceptable to Poles (Magdzik 2002a). This subtle distinction, and the reasons underlying it, are dealt with in some detail in Chapter 6. Fortunately the concept of 'obligation to society' is sufficient to ensure both individual and community protection without recourse to 'compulsion'.

The table on the next page represents the coverage figures for 2000.

The hepatitis B vaccination coverage calls for special mention. In the early 1990s, Poland had a very serious problem of hepatitis B infection, in fact the highest incidence (34 per 100 000) in Western and Central Europe, with young women being particularly affected due to their high exposure (both professionally and as patients) in healthcare settings. The strategy to combat this

Diphtheria/Tetanus	98.2%	(2nd year of life)
Pertussis	98.1%	(2nd year of life)
Poliomyelitis	98.2%	(2nd year of life)
Hepatitis B	99.3%	(2nd year of life)
Tuberculosis	95.5%	(newborn)
Measles	97.4%	(3rd year of life)
MMR	23.6%	(3rd year of life; *introduced only in 1996*)

[Source: PZH]

consisted of three components:

- rigorous training in infection control procedures for healthcare personnel
- the introduction of autoclaves for sterilisation
- an incremental programme of vaccination beginning with high-risk groups.

By 1999, the incidence rate of the disease had been brought down for the first time below 10 per 100 000 (Magdzik 2000b). The vaccination programme was introduced in 1994, and in 2000, as is shown above, 99.3% of children were vaccinated by their second year of life (Magdzik 2002b).

Uganda

Routine childhood immunisation in Uganda is, as in England, totally voluntary. Hence the country faces many of the same problems as England does in attempting to secure maximum coverage, along with some additional problems which are specific to the country. Very many agencies, including Non-Governmental Organisations (NGOs), are involved with the Government in these activities. The immunisation procedures are free of charge and are undertaken mainly by nurses and trained community vaccinators. The Uganda National Expanded Programme on Immunisation (UNEPI) is responsible for implementing the National Disease Control Department's programme relating to vaccine-preventable diseases, namely measles, poliomyelitis, pertussis, tetanus and diphtheria. It also provides the vaccines for immunisation against tuberculosis as part of the Childhood (under 5 years) Preventable Killer Diseases Programme (the programme responsible for tuberculosis prevention and control is the National Tuberculosis and Leprosy Programme, based in the Department of National Disease Control of the Ministry of Health). UNEPI's programme base is located at Entebbe, where its technical staff coordinate with the NGO sector on the establishment of standards, etc. but the Department of National Disease Control, in collaboration with other relevant technical departments, is responsible for policy development, overall coordination and guidance on immunisation. A National Immunisation Inter-Agency Coordinating Committee exists to provide support to the Government in immunisation planning and monitoring efforts. This committee is chaired by the Minister of Health in charge of primary health and contains representatives not only of the Ministry of Health's Clinical and Community Services and the National Council for Children, but also of the many participating partners including WHO, UNICEF, US Agency for International Development (USAID), Department for International Development (DFID) (UK), Uganda Red Cross and Rotary International. At the district level, the District Director of Health Services (DDHS) is responsible for the planning, management, coordination and monitoring of immunisation services with all agencies working at the district level. This question of working with all relevant agencies is a very important one at not only national but also lower levels, given the voluntary nature of the procedures and the very large number of agencies which are participating partners in the programme, and so every effort is made to involve political and other community leaders in the enterprise. The overall objective of UNEPI's programme is to attain the highest levels of coverage such that the target diseases are no longer of public health significance in the country. More specifically, national targets by the end of the 5-year period include:

- achieving coverage of children aged 12–23 months fully immunised from 44% to 80%
- increasing diphtheria/pertussis/tetanus (DPT) coverage from 55% to 80% (WHO 2001)
- increasing tetanus toxoid coverage of pregnant women from 42% to 80% (Health Sector Strategic Plan 2000/2001–2004/ 2005).

Routine childhood immunisation in Uganda has, until very recently, had a chequered history. Ugandan doctors themselves were in the forefront of developments in this field in that they were instrumental in launching Africa's first national immunisation campaign against poliomyelitis in 1967, despite severe financial constraints. However, by the 1970s, as a consequence of war and the disintegrating economy, immunisation suffered badly. For example, in 1973 over 70% of Ugandan children were immunised against tuberculosis, whereas by the end of the decade the figure was less than 10%. Measles was also, during this period, a major cause of child mortality; hospital deaths from this cause rose between 1970 and 1981 from 5% to 26%. After 1986, the programme was revitalised for a second time, and by the mid-1990s there had been significant achievements – 96% against tuberculosis, 85% for measles and 78% against poliomyelitis (Iliffe 1998). However, the coverage figures for these procedures had fallen to 77%, 56% and 53%, respectively, by the year 2000, alongside 72% for DPT1, 53% for DPT3 and 42% for maternal protection against tetanus (WHO/UNICEF 2002). This is the reason for the target figure of 80% aimed at in the 5-year Health Sector Strategic Plan.

Apart from the social dislocation consequent upon past war and civil disturbance, what other causes may there be for the decline in coverage evident in the second half of the 1990s? A useful index for this is the drop-out rate from DPT1 to DPT3 observed in more than 70% of the districts during this period (WHO 2001). The following have been suggested as possibly worthy of consideration.

1 Administrative decentralisation to the districts from 1995 meant that the latter received block grants for *all* services and immunisation was initially not necessarily seen as a priority (Lewis 2003).
2 Distrust of villagers over the safety of vaccination (possibly encouraged by those opposed to the Government who spread rumours that these are harmful procedures deliberately used by the Government to reduce the population); this could lead to children being hidden during immunisation campaigns (Bahá'í International Community 1999).
3 Some local communities may perhaps have forgotten the importance of completing the full doses, plus the fact that immunisation sessions may conflict with farming duties, especially during planting seasons (WHO 2001).
4 Technical problems affecting the functional cold chain system may impair the programme in certain districts.

It is noteworthy that the UNEPI programme, with all its inter-locking components, is concerned *inter alia* with relevant health education, timely delivery of immunisation services, and ensuring that all districts have adequate equipment and supplies to strengthen the capacity for cold chain maintenance at all levels. Ugandan Scouts play an important part in the support role by raising awareness of the importance of immunisation and by ensuring that appointments are kept; they can gain an Immunisation Proficiency Badge for these efforts. Also a dedicated outreach programme is to be put in place to serve the 'hard-to-reach' populations, and national or sub-national 'immunisation days' are declared from time to time as part of the campaigns against selected target diseases, for example poliomyelitis and measles. At the time of writing (February 2003), the most recent of these was on the weekend of 31 August/1 September 2002 and consisted of a sub-national immunisation day with the slogan:

'IMMUNISE!   DO NOT LET YOUR CHILD BE CRIPPLED!
TOGETHER, WE CAN KICK POLIO OUT OF UGANDA'

[This was appropriately illustrated by a picture of a young footballer giving the ball a vigorous kick high into the air.]

On these days, *all* children below five years of age were targetted, even though some might already have been immunised. The sub-national nature of the event related to the 18 districts which were selected for this purpose as they border countries with a high risk of poliovirus transmission (*The Monitor*, 31 August 2002); Uganda itself has not had a case of the disease since 1996.

It is reassuring to observe that these efforts are bearing fruit. Coverage is on the rise again; DPT3 coverage for 2002 is approximately 67% and measles coverage is estimated to be around 71% for the year (Lewis 2003).

Prevention of sexually-transmitted infections (STIs)

One other measure, in quite a different sphere, is worthy of mention in a chapter dealing with prevention. The recognition of the sexual mode of spread of HIV infection in the 1980s raised once more the use of condoms to reduce the risk of *all* sexually-transmitted infections; indeed the American Public Health Association's (APHA) current guidance recommends their use for the prevention of syphilis, gonorrhoea, and infection by chlamydia, herpes simplex, human papillomavirus and sexually-transmitted hepatitis B, in addition to HIV infection (APHA 2000). Mention has been made in Chapter 1 of the fact that psychological, social, religious and cultural factors can continue to constitute additional barriers to their use. It should perhaps be understood that it is not only in the developing world or in devout Roman Catholic communities that such factors may apply. In April 1986 the Chief Medical Officer of the Department of Health in London, Sir Donald Acheson, called a meeting of all district medical officers in England at which he urged them to promote educational messages in their districts concerning the modes of spread of HIV infection and the measures which could be taken to reduce the risk. Nevertheless, when the District Medical Officer of Coventry (the author) wished to mention condoms in a proposed feature in the local newspaper, the editor objected on the grounds that this would not be suitable for a family newspaper! It was only when, shortly afterwards, the Chief Medical Officer explained the concept of 'safer sex' in a television programme that the editor, and no doubt many others in his position, agreed that this was a word that could responsibly be used in advising the public. However, sensitivities concerning this issue clearly need to be handled delicately, as the following example shows.

In Malta in the mid-1980s the Department of Health in Valletta, in common with such establishments in many other countries, became concerned about the implications of HIV/AIDS. Measures were taken to eliminate the risk from transfusions of blood and blood products but for some time there was no discussion on the value of condoms in reducing the risk. The Roman Catholic Church exerts very considerable influence on political affairs in Malta and the general line of 'chastity before marriage and faithfulness within it' was the one which did not upset the Church. However, in the late 1980s there was wide distribution of a booklet, produced by the Chief Government Medical Officer, which mentioned not only condoms but also anal sex; this upset many people. In 1991 an international conference on HIV/AIDS was held in Malta, one outcome of which was the creation of a local advisory committee. A polemic then developed in the Press concerning condoms, with the Church arguing with several prominent public health doctors. The latter greatly welcomed the publicity as it had brought the matter out into the open. The controversy came to a head on World AIDS Day in 1993, when a poster was displayed showing a rolled-out condom. The opposition from the Church was such that the poster had to be withdrawn. Subsequently a QUANGO

('HANDS') was set up to to rally people who were HIV-positive into a self-help group and AIDS promotion issues were handed over to them. By the late 1990s, a special clinic for sexually-transmitted infections had been set up, run by an ex-British Army Maltese doctor, and this establishment sent out regular newsletters on HIV prevention to local doctors. The current position appears to be that there is a general understanding that, as long as these matters are discussed discreetly and sensibly, the Church will not react, and condom-dispensing machines are now available in night clubs, etc. (Falzon 2002).

In Uganda the approach to this preventive measure could not be more different. Early in 1986, following the creation of the Government's AIDS Control Programme, the new Minister of Health set up an AIDS surveillance sub-committee which began to organise both public education and the supply of protective condoms. A multisectoral approach was adopted by the Government in 1993 to create an atmosphere of political commitment to HIV/AIDS control. A policy of openness had been adopted early on with the emphasis on 'zero-grazing', i.e. faithfulness to one sexual partner. However, cultural resistance was initially strong; in 1993, for example, a survey carried out in two rural districts showed that only 3% of men regularly used condoms in spite of the promotional messages (Iliffe 1998). The policy of openness was also evident in the educational sphere. In 1986 the Ministry of Education and Sports launched an awareness campaign through media, theatre and school-based health education, thereby demonstrating that the education sector had a key role in the fight against AIDS, which was not to be treated as a 'health problem' pure and simple (Elimu 2001). The health promotional messages dealt with the wider aspects of behaviour – not just condoms – with good effect. For example a poster with the caption:

SUPPORT YOUR FRIENDS
HELP THEM TO REMAIN **AIDS** FREE

depicted three young women, two pulling back the third who was being enticed by an older man, a 'sugar daddy' who might infect her (*see* illustration). In fact, the average age of 'first sex' among young people of 15–19 (the age group considered to be most vulnerable to HIV infection) rose by two years between 2000 and 2002, a measure of a degree of success of the health promotional messages (Population Information Program 2002).

Since 1994 HIV infection levels have continued to decline (a

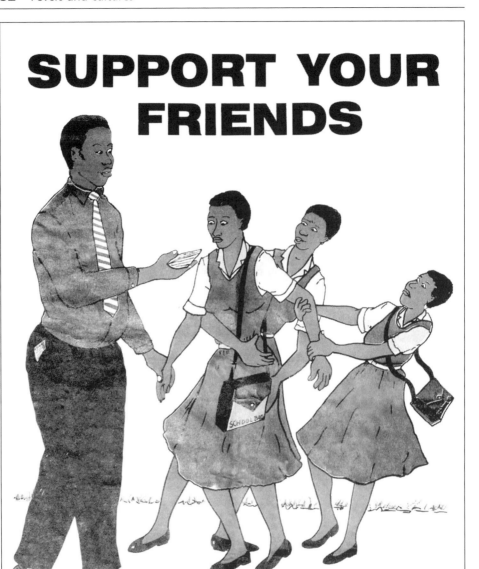

situation probably unique in sub-Saharan Africa) and these achievements have been attributed to the multisectoral approach to HIV/AIDS prevention and control spearheaded by the Government, and matched by the positive response of communities in sexual behaviour change. Moves towards such change are aided by the fact that the social climate in Uganda is such that open discussions on sexual matters are possible without embarrassment; the relevance of this factor, with appropriate examples, is explored a little in Chapter 6. To maintain this health gain, the Health Sector Strategic Plan includes the following among its objectives.

1 To increase and sustain male condom use from 50% to 75% in rural areas, and sustain the rate in urban areas at or above the current rate of 80%.
2 To increase female condom use to about 25% for both urban and rural areas.
3 To increase HIV voluntary counselling and testing services.

CHAPTER 5

Control

Control measures can be directed *against* both the source of infection and the path of transmission and *towards* protecting persons exposed to it. In this account, the latter does *not* include protection against vaccine-preventable diseases as the principles have already been covered in Chapter 4; the focus here is mainly, but not solely, on actions taken to deal with human sources of infection, i.e. *cases*, *contacts* or *carriers*. Although in practice most people are probably motivated to be cooperative in public health activities designed to prevent the spread of infection (provided that these measures are explained adequately), laws exist in many countries to ensure, as far as practicable, that irresponsible behaviour does not put individuals, groups or communities at risk. This chapter concerns itself with the key public health *medical** activities which can, if necessary, be enforced by law.

Cases of disease are likely to come to attention by formal notification by clinicians or reporting by laboratory microbiologists as part of the surveillance system illustrated in its simplest form in Figure 2.2 (*see* p 20). Figure 5.1 shows a simplified model of transmission of infectious disease. Notification of certain infectious diseases is a legal requirement in most countries. In England clinicians receive a modest fee for notifying a case, but in France the attitude can be summed up as 'One does not reward someone for merely complying with the law!' Notification by telephone, in the case of certain specified infectious diseases, allows the most rapid public health response. This is most relevant where the disease is a serious or potentially fatal one, the incubation period or latent period is short, close contacts are at high risk and rapid intervention can be life-saving; meningococcal infection and diphtheria, for example, meet all four criteria.

In some countries telephone notification in such situations is

---

* This work is concerned primarily with the work of medical personnel in this field.

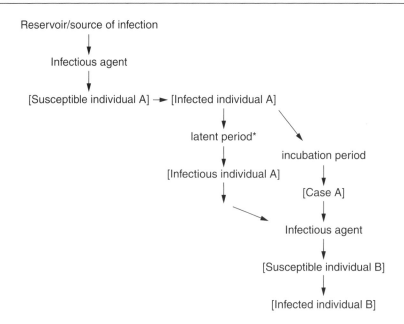

Figure 5.1 Simplified model of transmission.
* *Illustration of significance of latent period*: The time spent in the infected state before becoming infectious. This may be shorter than the incubation period, as in hepatitis A, for example, and therefore of considerable public health importance.

mandatory; in others it depends essentially on a good rapport between the public health physician and local clinicians, a situation which can invariably be improved by positive action.

Control of infection from *cases* is mostly straightforward, whether the patient is at home or in hospital. Chemotherapy, plus varying degrees of isolation and/or barrier nursing in the latter location, may be called for if, for example, the patient is suffering from a highly contagious or virulent infection, has a positive tuberculosis sputum or has an infection transmitted by direct or indirect contact with faeces. Outside hospital, advice on appropriate behaviour to avoid spread of infection may be necessary. However, rarely, isolation has to be enforced, in a situation where an infectious patient knowingly and recklessly puts others at risk and cannot be persuaded to take reasonable precautions; open tuberculosis is the usual disease in which this course of action may be required. With regard to certain diseases, it is usual to follow up *contacts* of notified cases to ensure the identification of all potentially infectious persons and to offer, where appropriate, protection to individuals by chemoprophylaxis (e.g. isoniazid for tuberculosis contacts and erythromycin for diphtheria contacts). Preventing the spread of infection from *healthy carriers* frequently concerns food handlers and, if the public health authority has been made aware of such a situation, negotiated financial arrangements may be considered so that the individual does not suffer loss of earnings as a result of remaining off work until free from the risk of spreading infection. The sequential outbreaks of typhoid in the wake of the cook Mary Mallon in nineteenth and twentieth century New York demonstrate the devastating effects of failure to be able to do this:

Federspiel's book, The Ballad of Typhoid Mary *(1984), tells the story. Born in Graubünden, in Switzerland, Maria Caduff (she assumed the name of Mary Mallon later) arrived in New York as a 12-year-old immigrant with no skills other than her professed ability to cook. Thereafter in both hotels and private homes in and around New York, for a period of nearly 40 years, she worked as a cook, causing repeated outbreaks of typhoid among those who consumed her dishes. Shrewdly moving on from place to place at just the right moment, she was able to evade investigation by the authorities until finally tracked down by the New York City Board of Health and, on the basis of typhoid bacilli having been identified in a stool specimen, she was isolated in Riverside Hospital on North Brother Island in Long Island Sound, where she died in 1938, eight years after a cerebral haemorrhage. Mary always claimed that she had never at any time knowingly suffered from typhoid fever; this could certainly have been the truth, in which case she was probably the most dangerous infectious disease carrier in recorded history and truly deserved the nickname 'Typhoid Mary'.*

Nearer to home, in the 1960s while the author was learning his craft as a public health physician, he had his first experience of finding a typhoid carrier. A young child admitted to hospital died of a cerebral abscess; most unusually, the organism isolated from the lesion turned out to be *Salmonella typhi* and phage-typing showed it to be a strain found in a particular location in the Caribbean. The child had never been outside England and no-one in the family was found on investigation to be carrying the organism. More detailed investigation revealed that the child had been day-minded in a small group by an unregistered child minder, an elderly lady who originated from that same Caribbean location. She had no history of ever having had the disease but stool examination showed that she was excreting the organism. Many attempts were made to rid her of the carrier state by treatment in the local infectious disease hospital but these were unsuccessful and so she was given detailed advice on scrupulous personal hygiene and advised not to undertake any further child-minding work, nor to cook for others.

Paths of transmission

Control over *paths of transmission* involves a wide range of activities which depend on whether they are:

- *direct* or
- *indirect*.

Direct transmission

Now that contagious skin infections are readily controllable by antibiotic treatment, the most important conditions spread by direct contact are sexually transmitted diseases. As the author's teaching commitments have included countries where the populations have been almost totally Roman Catholic, he has found it helpful to refer to the guidance offered by the American Public Health Association (APHA 1995):

> '... safer sexual practices, i.e. mutual monogamy with a non-infected partner, avoiding multiple sexual partners or casual or anonymous sex and consistent use of condoms with all partners not known to be free from a sexually-transmitted disease.'

However, the concept of 'safe sex' *at a population level* is open to question. The view has been put forward (Alcabes 2000) that although condom use may be effective on a 'per contact' basis, only if 'coverage' of the population is very high is there any real community benefit. His contention is that even in a population with, for example, an extremely high HIV prevalence, one would have to convince at least half of the population to use condoms *every time* in order to bring about a measurable reduction in HIV incidence, and that in low prevalence populations it would be virtually impossible to make a dent in the incidence in this way. These reservations are based on the belief that most people don't use condoms, and that even most of those who do, don't most of the time.

Indirect transmission

This represents a major area for public health control by *scientific*, *technical* and *educational* methods rather than by medical activities involving, as it does, such diverse measures as:

- purification of public water supplies
- pasteurisation of milk
- hygienic food practices
- chemical treatment of water in cooling-towers
- screening of blood and blood products
- education of injecting drug-misusers
- protection against insect bites (in warmer climates).

It would not be practicable, in a book of this kind, to try to cover such a complex field, although some examples have been briefly mentioned elsewhere because of their profound public health significance, for example Legionnaires' disease in the United States, the 'three affairs of contaminated blood' in France, and brucellosis in Malta.

At first sight, air-borne transmission would appear to be an appropriate area for attention but, apart from common sense precautions to be taken by persons when coughing or sneezing, and special ventilation arrangements in hospital isolation units, there are very few examples of successful or acceptable practices for destruction of organisms in the air, for example by chemical aerosols or ultraviolet radiation. [One rare exception has been the use of vaporised formaldehyde for terminal disinfection of textile mills contaminated with the anthrax bacillus, the spores of the organism having remained viable in hides imported from countries where the disease is still endemic among animals. Hence 'wool-sorters' disease' – one descriptive name for pulmonary anthrax. This may, of course, become a live issue once more in the light of bioterrorism threats.] If one thinks of potentially serious air-borne infections such as tuberculosis or diphtheria it is significant that protection depends essentially on control of the infectious source, for example by isolation, alongside relevant host-protection measures such as immunisation procedures, active or passive, the latter possibly combined with protective chemotherapy.

Figure 2.2 (*see* p 20) showed how surveillance maintains a lookout for trouble in the form of cases, outbreaks or epidemics of infectious disease. However, it has an ongoing function to assess

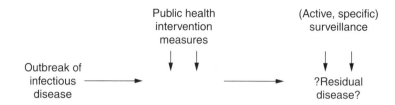

Figure 5.2 Control and surveillance.

the effectiveness of whatever control measures have been implemented. In this latter case, the surveillance has to be both active and specific in that the public health authority has to actively seek information relating to a specific infection (Figure 5.2).

The following relates, as mentioned earlier, to the key public health *medical* activities aimed at the control of communicable diseases in the six countries.

England

The pandemic of bubonic plague was probably the first spur to concerted action aimed at communicable disease control in England, as in many other European countries. By 1346 the Black Death had spread westward from the Black Sea to the thriving Adriatic and Mediterranean ports and, crossing Europe, it reached England two years later by way of a ship carrying fugitives from a terrible outbreak in Calais to the small Dorset port of Melcombe Regis (Hirst 1953). In the same year, the Venetian Republic had taken an initiative in detaining and observing suspect ships, followed rapidly by Ragusa (Dubrovnik) and Marseille. Maritime quarantine of this type had no reasonable possibility of succeeding as there was no knowledge at that time of the role that the rat played in the chain of infection, let alone that of the rat flea or the plague bacillus. Even much later, in 1663, when regulations decreed that plague-infested vessels approaching London were not to be allowed beyond Gravesend, where they were maintained for 30 days, this did not subsequently prevent the Great Plague in London two years later.

It was not until the eighteenth century that quarantine, as part of a package of control measures, may possibly have protected England against the disease. Plague, having disappeared from the whole of Europe by 1683, reappeared in Marseille from Africa in

1720. The Government, alarmed at the possibility of its reintroduction into England, commissioned Richard Mead, a Fellow of both the College of Physicians and the Royal Society, to produce 'guidelines' to protect the health of the nation. Mead's prompt response was to produce the classic *A Short Discourse Concerning Pestilential Contagion and the Methods to be Used to Prevent it*. He clearly saw as the top priority the need to prevent plague from entering England in the first place:

> '*As it is a satisfaction to know that the plague is not a native of our country, so this is likewise an encouragement to the utmost diligence in finding out means to keep ourselves clear from it. This is provided by the established method of obliging ships that come from infected places to perform quarantine*' (Mead 1720).

In the event, plague did not spread from France to England but, as one cannot say with certainty whether Mead's advice played a key role in this, perhaps equal or even greater benefit was gained from the fact that his *Short Discourse* covered the entire gamut of public health action including case-finding, isolation, abatement of overcrowding, etc., thus setting a pattern for future control measures which applies up to the present day.

It was, almost certainly, the subsequent *failure* of stringent quarantine to prevent the arrival of cholera in England in 1831 which triggered off the establishment of what might be regarded as the first locally-based public health service in the country. It brought into being, within three years of the onset of this epidemic, more than 1200 local boards of health, locally elected and vested with the duty of protecting the health of the people in the area.

In the following 10 years in the wake of the cholera epidemic, the famous report of Sir Edwin Chadwick, Chairman of the Poor Law Commission, on the 'sanitary condition of the labouring population' persuaded the Government that sanitation was a public question (Poor Law Commissioners 1842). Chadwick was, in fact, under pressure to cut the costs of 'public relief' under the Poor Law and was working on the assumption that prevention would be cheaper than relief, particularly the prevention of the death from infectious disease of the male breadwinner who would thereby leave a dependent family (Lewis 1991). His report proved conclusively that disease was associated with insanitary environmental conditions due to polluted water, poor drainage and a lack of means of removing refuse from houses and streets. The fact that he believed that such disease was due to unwholesome exhalations from decaying animal and vegetable matter (the miasma theory) was irrelevant. His recommended remedies, drainage, street and house cleansing, by means of supplies of water and improved sewerage, were effective. Although he specified the key role of civil engineering in effecting these improvements, he accepted the need for a medical input in specifying the nature, location and likely course of the disease:

> 'That for the promotion of the means necessary to prevent disease, it would be good economy to appoint a district medical officer, independent of private practice, and with securities of special qualifications, and (with) responsibilities to initiate sanitary measures and reclaim the execution of the law' (Poor Law Commissioners 1842).

Thus communicable disease was seen as an essentially local problem requiring a local solution, the medical element of which was taken up first by the City of Liverpool with the appointment of Dr Andrew Duncan as Officer of Health in 1847 and Dr John Simon as Medical Officer of Health (MOH) of the City of London in the following year. Six years later, shrewd observations by a London physician, Dr John Snow, established a direct connection between 500 fatal cases of cholera and the pump in Broadwick Street, Soho, which supplied their water. His recommendation to the authorities that the pump should be shut off constituted such an important milestone in communicable disease control that a John Snow Society has been formed to commemorate his work. The appointment of MOHs from 1847 onwards firmly established the model of a medically-led, locally-based public health service, soon to profit from the development of scientific bacteriology based on the work of Pasteur and Koch. It is interesting to speculate whether, had quarantine *not* failed to provide the expected protection, a locally-based public health service would have developed quite so quickly in England, a service whose general principles continued until 1974.

Chapter 3 referred to the fact that the MOH post had been abolished as a casualty of the 1974 NHS reorganisation, in the erroneous belief by the Government that 'infectious diseases had been virtually eliminated as health problems'. The point in that chapter was made in relation to the lack of development of surveillance but, in fact, it was in the sphere of communicable disease *control* that the public – and the politicians – noted the deficiencies. The replacement post for the control of communicable disease locally, the Medical Officer for Environmental Health (MOEH) in each district, had to contend with a number of difficulties and frustrations:

- lack of direct support, from medical, nursing and environmental health staff
- a tendency for their activities to be marginalised
- a feeling of professional isolation.

Against this background it was unfortunate for the country to have to cope with emerging infectious diseases in the 1970s such as:

1973	Rotaviral enteritis
1976	Cryptosporidiosis
	Legionnaires' disease
	Lassa fever
1977	Campylobacter food poisoning
	Ebola-Marburg diseases

along with two outbreaks of smallpox (one in London, one in Birmingham), even before the 1980s brought such alarming newcomers as toxic shock syndrome, *E. coli* 0157:H7 haemorrhagic colitis, HIV/AIDS and hepatitis C.

The public inquiries arising from the two major outbreaks, of *Salmonella* food poisoning in 1984 and Legionnaires' disease in the following year, referred to in Chapter 3, led in due course to the Acheson Committee's report *Public Health in England* (HMSO 1988). This resulted in the abolition of the unsatisfactory MOEH post and its replacement by the post soon to be known as the CCDC, the latter to have executive responsibility for the surveillance, prevention and control of communicable disease and infection at local (i.e. DHA, and subsequently PCT) level.

At the same time the report drew attention to the fact that some of the problems arose from the complexity of legislation on communicable disease control and from misunderstanding about its interpretation. The Public Health (Control of Disease) Act 1984, together with its corresponding regulations, in particular the Public Health (Infectious Diseases) Regulations 1988, were largely consolidating measures and many of the provisions in this legislation dated from as far back as the late nineteenth century. A key recommendation was that there should be a review of the law to clarify which infectious diseases should continue to be notified, whether there should be different categories depending on the urgency of action required, and what powers were needed by the CCDC to restrict the movement or activities of individuals or to invoke environmental control powers.

To date (February 2003), although a variety of working groups have reviewed the law, no new legislation for this purpose has yet appeared on the Statute Book. The lack of progress on this front has continued to give cause for concern. The most recent major expression of this is found in a report by the Nuffield Trust for Research and Policy Studies *The State of Communicable Disease Law* (Monaghan 2002). This argues that the public health legal framework has been neglected and that the law dealing with the control of communicable disease is inadequate, outdated and in need of reform. It emphasises that the potential threats from infectious diseases are diverse and that, in the aftermath of September 11 2001, the possibility of bioterrorism has reinforced the need for an effective strategy to combat the threat of new and emerging, as well as existing, diseases. It suggests that new legislation should move the legal authority to the new Health Protection Agency (briefly described in Appendix 2) which should be given a specific statutory duty to provide a communicable disease control service to every local district.

However, the existing legislation gives the CCDC the authority, for example:

- to receive notifications
- to require an individual to submit to medical examination (including microbiological and radiological)
- to discontinue work (e.g. a food handler)
- to be admitted to hospital and detained there (e.g. a recalcitrant patient with infectious tuberculosis).

The constraints upon the individual are to be used only in circumstances where they are necessary to prevent the spread of infection. There are built-in safeguards, such as the involvement of the local authority (usually one of its solicitors) and/or a Justice of the Peace, which ensure that the individual is not, for example, inappropriately deprived of his or her liberty. Curiously enough the CCDC's authority to receive notifications applies only to clinicians. Reporting by laboratory microbiologists is, by some quirk of the law, quite informal although it tends by virtue of traditional professionalism to be comprehensive (Figure 5.3).

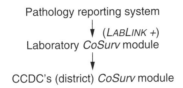

Pathology reporting system

(*LABLINK +*)

Laboratory *CoSurv* module

CCDC's (district) *CoSurv* module

Figure 5.3   Reporting by laboratory microbiologists.

Within the limits of the out-of-date legislation as far as authority is concerned, the role of the CCDC is worth examining in some detail. The fact that the first initial stands for 'consultant' has considerable significance. For the first time an overt attempt was made to bring this post into line with the status (and salary) of that of a clinical consultant, with its implications of *professional autonomy*. This, along with the fact that the post was to be a truly specialist one, focusing on communicable disease control exclusively, was intended to accord it the proper status as a medical specialty and this was reflected in the length of specialised postgraduate training (at least four years) and the nature of the appointment procedure. The Advisory Appointments Committee was based on the hospital consultant model, with clinicians and the local university represented, along with health authority and local authority members and two assessors appointed by the Faculty of Public Health Medicine. [If microbiology candidates were to be interviewed, one of the assessors was to be appointed by the Royal College of Pathologists.] The significance of the Committee being so formidable and the interview so rigorous was that any successful candidate (who since 1996 would have acquired the Certificate of Completion of Specialist Training) was deemed to be competent enough to fulfil the role in an autonomous manner – what might be regarded as the 'epidemiological' equivalent of clinical autonomy.

Although the specialised resources of the CDSC were to be made available to assist the CCDC in for example a major outbreak, *this could only be at the CCDC's request*. Additionally, the CCDC had to inform the Chief Medical Officer of the Department of Health, and also the CDSC, only in the case of *serious* outbreaks, or those which might have wider than local significance or which presented unusual features in terms of scale, complexity or potential threat to the health of the population (Figure 5.4). It is worth making this 'cultural' point as it reflects an aversion to centralisation and professional direction, which is a cultural characteristic of English practice in this field.

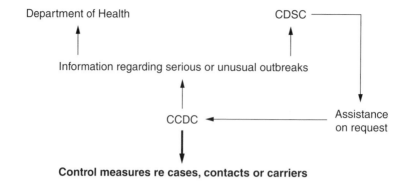

Figure 5.4   Role of the CCDC in *control* of communicable disease.

In order to investigate the extent to which the arrangements recommended in *Public Health in England* had been implemented, the Chief Medical Officer of the Department of Health commissioned a survey of all districts in England (referred to in Chapter 3). This showed that the CCDC role had been widely established but that the post-holders were experiencing two main difficulties, namely lack of resources and problems in attempting to discharge their duties within the framework of the existing law (Pollock *et al.* 1991). These problems were felt especially in the London area. Reference was made in Chapter 3 to the benefits to the CCDCs in London from the pan-London surveillance project. However, these CCDCs made it clear that they would not be agreeable to such a unit, or a parallel one, having any functions in the *control* of communicable disease as they felt that such an arrangement would encroach upon their statutory responsibilities (Pollock 1993).

Note: Brief mention is made in Appendix 2 of the fact that, under the provisions of the Government's report *Getting Ahead of the Curve: a strategy for combating infectious diseases (including other aspects of health protection)* (DoH 2002), a new Health Protection Agency is to become operational in April 2003. Although the mention in Appendix 2 relates to the proposed new arrangements for national communicable disease surveillance, the implications for the organisation of communicable disease *control* are quite profound. The new agency is to operate through a number of divisions, including a Division of Field Services which is to be staffed mainly by existing CCDCs, so that the latter will be brought into a new organisation with a wide range of specialist expertise, in which communicable disease control will become part of the wider health protection function.

United States

In Chapter 3 brief reference was made to the fact that, arising out of the Constitution, an important question is that of the relative powers of state and federal government, the latter having been conceived as one of limited powers. According to the Tenth Amendment, any powers *not* given to the federal government remain with the states. Such powers, including authority over matters of public health, were left to the individual states as 'states' rights' (Fee 1997). Therefore each state has its own written constitution which plays a key role in determining the law of that state; it has a full set of legal institutions, a governor, executive agencies and staff, and represents the basic law-making unit, submitting only to superior federal law (Clark and Ansay 1992). This means that the state is 'autonomous' with regard to *inter alia* the control of communicable diseases. State reporting requirements, as pointed out in Chapter 3, vary with regard to diseases to be reported, time-frames for reporting, agencies receiving reports, persons required to report, and penalties for not reporting (Chorba *et al.* 1989). (The situation post-September 2001 has, of course, changed significantly in the wake of the anthrax attacks through the US mail, as explained in Chapter 6.)

Once more regarding the State of Oklahoma as *illustrative* for this purpose (rather than representative, because of the diversity of the states), it is the State's responsibility to decide which diseases should be on the reportable list but this 'autonomy' is influenced by the fact that there is a general professional consensus within the Council of State and Territorial Epidemiologists on which diseases should at least form the core of such lists in *every* state. The Oklahoma State Department of Health is accountable to the State Board of Health and is headed by a Commissioner of Health assisted by five Deputy Commissioners, each responsible for one service division. Within one of the latter lies the Epidemiology Service headed by the State Epidemiologist who, in turn, is assisted by the Director of the Communicable Diseases Section (a senior medical epidemiologist) who is in day-to-day charge of communicable disease control for the State as a whole.

Formal reporting by a physician or microbiologist, required by law, is made either direct to the Director of the Infectious Diseases

Section or to the county health department of the area in which the case has occurred. If the latter, the details must be passed on to the State as soon as possible so that the director has all the information required to institute whatever control measures are considered appropriate. Laboratory reporting has been found to be more dependable than that from physicians but the latter do not tend to be actually penalised for failure to report as it is felt that this would be counterproductive (Quinlisk 1998). On behalf of the State Legislature or Department of Health, the director can enforce other control measures such as exclusion of a person from work or admission to the State Hospital to prevent spread of infection, the latter generally with regard to infectious tuberculosis.

The director has the support of a small team of non-medical epidemiologists who are able to constitute a 24-hour 'on-call' rota so that each notification is passed to the duty epidemiologist for advice on necessary action at local level by the (mainly nursing) staff of the relevant county health department. The Director, as a senior specialised public health physician, is always available for consultation in cases of difficulty. The existence and routine use of a manual of control policies and procedures, prepared by the Director on behalf of the whole state, simplify problem solving at local level and help to ensure acceptable standards.

Each of the counties within the State has a county health department but these are staffed by personnel whose salaries are paid by the State and who are therefore really outposted State employees. The two exceptions are the counties of Oklahoma City and Tulsa which, because of their size (populations of over a million and 360 000 respectively), for day-to-day purposes are almost completely independent of the State Department of Health, each having its own Board of Health, Medical Director and supporting staff of epidemiologists and nurses. The professional and organisational relationships between these two counties and the State are such that the former routinely use the State's manual of control procedures, and in the event of a major outbreak the State would assist by informally seconding appropriate staff. [The principle of relative independence is more common in for example New York State, where many of the counties are virtually coterminous with large cities such as Buffalo, Rochester and Albany, many having their own medical directors. The guiding principle on this matter in New York State is that if a (presumably large) county wishes to have its own relatively independent medical director, then it has to meet the cost of this arrangement (Morse 1993).]

The federal involvement in communicable disease control was, until September 11 2001, minimal. Oklahoma State regarded the role of the relevant federal organisation – CDC Atlanta – as 'advisory' only but the latter had no difficulty in, for example, routinely obtaining the weekly electronic reports from the State as, on behalf of the federal government, it has traditionally funded around 80% of the costs of the State's activities in the surveillance, prevention and control of communicable diseases. The general post-September 11 situation is covered in Chapter 6.

France

As mentioned in Chapter 3, all formal requirements with regard to the control of communicable disease in France, in addition to those for surveillance and prevention, are to be found in *Art. Lois 1–18* of the *Code de la Santé Publique*. As Cairns and McKeon (1995) have pointed out, the codified system illustrates a characteristically French approach towards the law and the solving of legal problems. It is based on rationalism and is essentially deductive, starting from broad principles which are then applied to individual cases; this approach is examined a little in Chapter 6. By virtue of the laws of decentralisation of 1983, promised by President Mitterand in his 1981 election campaign, the level of authority for the control of the diseases notified is the département (Desenclos 1998a). At that level, within the Direction Départementale des Affaires Sanitaires et Sociales (DDASS), the medical official with the responsibility for control measures, previously mentioned in Chapters 3 and 4 in connection with surveillance and routine childhood immunisation respectively, is the Médecin Inspecteur de Santé Publique (MISP) (Ecole Nationale de Santé Publique 1995). This individual is by no means the exact equivalent of the English CCDC, but rather similar to an English Director of Public Health whose duties *include* those of the CCDC, as is shown below.

Unlike the CCDC, the MISP is not a specialist in communicable disease control, but rather a generic public health physician in the widest possible sense. For example, under 'Fields of Intervention', the MISP's training has to include cancer, cardiovascular diseases, invalidity, handicap, drug addiction, mental health and health of prisoners, in addition to communicable disease control. Furthermore these eight topics together form just one half of the module entitled 'Prevention and Health Promotion', itself being only one of three sections in that part of the course covering 'Conception and Implementation of Health Policy', during the academic year as a stagiaire (trainee) public health medical official at the Ecole Nationale de la Santé Publique (ENSP) in Rennes (*Le Métier de Médecin Inspecteur de Santé Publique et la Formation* 1997).

The use of the term 'official' is deliberate in that, in the relative absence of any very specialised expertise in the field of communicable disease control, the measures which the MISP has to take following the notification of a case are largely prescribed by circulars which have been issued by Central Government, after advice from the relevant professional bodies such as the Conseil Supérieur d'Hygiène Publique (CSHPF) and the Haut Comité de Santé Publique (HCSP). Additionally, although the situation has been changing rapidly with the coming into being of the Réseau National de Santé Publique and more recently the Institut de Veille Sanitaire, there has in the past been a tradition of the MISP both reporting to and being guided by the medical epidemiologist civil servants of the Bureau des Maladies Transmissibles within the Direction Générale de la Santé, on the management of any outbreak. Thus the MISP does not have anything corresponding to the considerable degree of local professional autonomy enjoyed by the CCDC. In fact, whether operating traditionally under the professional guidance of the Bureau des Maladies Transmissibles or, more recently, that of the Institut de Veille Sanitaire, the MISP appears to be functioning almost as an 'outposted' medical official of Central Government, rather than as an autonomous local professional.

Also, the MISP does not appear to have much in the way of formal authority to require action in certain local situations, for example for the protection of public health:

- to order the medical examination of a case, carrier or contact of a notifiable infectious disease
- to have someone admitted to hospital and detained there
- to exclude someone, e.g. a food handler, from work.

However, in the last-mentioned of these situations a doctor employed by the company or by a local cabinet de médecine de travail (occupational health agency) can issue a certificate of unfitness for those particular duties along with a request that alternative work be offered. If there are no such tasks, the employee is sent home (without salary) and has to depend on his or her family doctor to arrange for sick leave, until bacteriological evidence of freedom of risk allows the occupational health physician to certify fitness to return to work. Similarly, *Section III Art. Loi 17* of the

Code de la Santé Publique states that in an emergency situation, i.e. an epidemic or other imminent danger to public health, the prefect of the département or the mayor of the commune can order the execution of certain health measures *if not in conflict with all other rights* (my italics). The interpretation of this text is open for discussion but in reality such an emergency situation would only be declared in major disasters such as a large outbreak of plague (De Valk 2002).

Malta

In Chapter 4 mention was made of the fact that the French occupation, although comparatively brief, had had the effect of significantly influencing Maltese public health legislative aspects of routine childhood immunisation. The same can be said for the effect which the Code Napoléon had on the approach to communicable disease *control*. However the Prevention of Disease Ordinance, referred to in Chapter 4, is currently (February 2003) in the process of being replaced by a new Public Health Act, and a new Infectious Disease Notification Certificate has been brought in as an interim measure which, it is hoped, will be more user-friendly to clinicians. This new Public Health Act was due to be presented to the Maltese Parliament for the first reading soon after the summer 2002 recess; interestingly, the intention is to move the legal situation in the direction of English law in these matters (Amato-Gauci 2002).

Nevertheless the Prevention of Disease Ordinance (1908 as amended) is still valid and currently governs the formality of control procedures. As mentioned in Chapter 3, communicable disease control is undertaken by three MOHs (perhaps paradoxically a *British* title until 1974, in spite of the French influence on the law). One is reponsible for Valletta and the South East of the main island (including the port and airport), one for the North West (including, from Ta' Xbiex through Sliema to Mellieha Bay, the main concentration of hotels, camping sites, restaurants, bars and snackbars), and a third for the separate island of Gozo (essentially a holiday resort). All three work from the same central office in the Department of Public Health in Msida and are accountable to the Principal Medical Officer who is also responsible for disease surveillance for the Maltese Islands. This allows all four to work as a team and – especially important – *enables surveillance and control to be very closely integrated*. One unusual feature of the Malta situation, noted by the author while teaching at the Medical School there, is that many local doctors, mainly general practitioners but also some junior hospital doctors, are keen to acquire a postgraduate qualification in public health. This, apparently, is at least partly related to their wish to obtain or retain part-time Government appointments in the Public Health Service, but almost certainly also indicates a genuine interest in the subject.

The Prevention of Disease Ordinance conveys an impression of considerable formality, placing the responsibility for notification of a case, for example, on not only the medical practitioner but also the 'head of the family and in his default the nearest relative of the patient'. Similarly, the MOH is given wide powers, for example:

- to restrict the movements, including suspension from work, of a person suspected of being capable of spreading disease
- to order that a patient actually suffering from such a disease be isolated or given medical treatment or both
- to order that such a patient has periodic medical examinations and investigations as may be deemed necessary to ascertain such a person's freedom from infection
- to order that, if need be, and with the support of a second medical practitioner and the agreement of a magistrate, such a patient may be admitted to hospital and detained there so long as infected.

Penalties for 'disobeying or preventing any other person from obeying any such order' are severe; in certain circumstances the MOH can involve the police to assist in the achievement of these objectives. Perhaps because of the importance of farming to the Maltese economy, the history of brucellosis in the country, and in more recent years the growth of tourism, those parts of the Prevention of Disease Ordinance concerned with the prevention and control of infectious disease affecting animals have assumed particular significance.

Poland

In Chapter 3, the flow of information for surveillance purposes was diagramatically set out, i.e. from the clinician to the dyrektor, medical director of the relevant local powiat health/epidemiological station (the stacja sanitarno-epidemiologiczna or sanepid), thence onwards to the regional województwo level, finally being relayed to the Department of Epidemiology at the National Institute of Hygiene (PZH) for overall monitoring and feedback. However, it is very much at the local powiat level that the actual control activities are carried out; this state of affairs has certainly been strengthened by the moves towards greater delegation of authority in recent years (Magdzik 2000a).

Using as an illustration the powiat of Żyrardów (an industrial town of some 76 000 population, about 20 miles from Warsaw) the dyrektor of the local sanepid unit possesses an additional qualification in epidemiology and exercises two complementary sets of responsibilities.

1 Powiatowy inspektor sanitarny (local public health physician, similar to the English CCDC and not, as might be imagined from the title, the equivalent of an English environmental health officer).
2 Director/manager of the sanepid, including its bacteriological laboratory, a health educator, and nursing staff for assistance with epidemiological duties and vaccination work, i.e. routine activities such as the annual influenza drive and 'one-off' courses of injections, e.g. for persons bitten by animals in situations where the risk of rabies is significant.

This last-mentioned situation illustrates one aspect of cooperation between the dyrektor at local powiat level and the Veterinary Laboratory Service which is provided at the level of the województwo. [When the author was visiting the National Veterinary Research Institute in Puławy in 2001, he commented that this public health/veterinary cooperation appeared to be much better developed in Poland than in England and was given the smiling reply 'Wait till you have endemic rabies in your country!'] A brief description of the National Programme of Rabies Control is outlined at the end of this section.

The legal authority given to the dyrektor for the control of communicable diseases locally is considerable. The Act of Communicable Diseases and Infections (Ustawa o Chorobach Zakaźnych i Zakażeniach) and the Act of Tuberculosis Control (Ustawa o Zwalczaniu Gruźlicy) authorise, if need be:

● bacteriological investigations of a person suspected of suffering from a notifiable infectious disease
● exclusion of a person (e.g. a food handler) from work if relevant infection is suspected, until confirmed clear

- hospitalisation of a sputum-positive tuberculosis case and compulsory treatment until non-infectious, followed by supervision and surveillance after being discharged from hospital.

In addition to these pieces of basic legislation, there are a number of instructions, decrees, communiqués and dispositions of the Health Minister which contribute to the authority of the dyrektor who can, if necessary, call upon the police or City Guard to enforce these actions, especially with regard to suspending a person from work. However, such situations are very rare as Polish people are more and more conscious of the menace of infectious diseases and the wish to avoid threats to their health and to that of their families and the local community (as explained in Chapter 4 with regard to routine childhood immunisation). Control of HIV/AIDS is not the responsibility of the dyrektor at powiat level; instead this is dealt with at the regional – województwo – level so that, for example, as far as the powiat of Żyrardów is concerned (and, for that matter, 36 other powiats) by the dyrektor of the sanepid of Mazowieckie, the region which also includes Warsaw (Korycka 2002b).

Although the first Polish HIV infections, in the mid-1980s, appeared to have been among male homosexuals, by 1993 or 1994 the epidemic was clearly driven by injecting drug misuse; by that time, 70% of Polish AIDS cases were reportedly occurring in drug injectors. The central feature of the AIDS epidemic was the injection of homemade or locally-produced drugs, especially kompot. This is an opiate extracted from the dried stems and heads of poppies, using chloroform or acetone, in the home kitchen – a discovery originally made by chemists in Gdańsk as far back as 1976. The problem has been especially marked in Upper Silesia, a part of the country where unemployment is especially high. Consideration has recently been given to the practicalities of endeavouring to ensure that every injection is accomplished with a sterile syringe. In this connection, considerable doubt has been cast on the belief that 'sharing syringes is a valued part of the culture of drug misuse' as recent research has shown that no drug injector has declined to use a sterile syringe when this has been offered (Alcabes 2000). However, the cost and availability of syringes, general risk-taking behaviour among drug users, punitive laws and social stigma surrounding drug misuse are many of the factors which make the future spread of HIV infection difficult to predict (Balińska 2000). In 1998, the number of notified and registered AIDS cases was quite stable, but some increase of HIV infection was observed. The quality of collected epidemiological data has depended – partly – on easy access to HIV testing, completeness of data, and diagnosis of AIDS indicator diseases by definitive methods (Szata 2000).

The syringe is also an important vehicle in both hepatitis B and C. In Chapter 4, mention was made of the introduction of autoclaves in healthcare settings, alongside a rigorous programme of training in infection control for healthcare personnel and an incremental programme of vaccination, which together were so successful in tackling the serious problem of hepatitis B infection. Interestingly, an evaluation of hepatitis C surveillance in Poland in 1998 suggested that exposure in healthcare settings might account for a high proportion of new cases of hepatitis C infection. It was recommended that this finding should be confirmed in analytical studies (Mazurek *et al.* 2002). [Some early follow-up work, i.e. a case control study, has provided evidence that, during 1998, hospitalisation, specifically surgical procedures and injections, had in fact played an important role in the transmission of hepatitis C infection (Mazurek *et al.* in press) and so the replacement of dry-heat sterilisers by autoclaves and the staff training activities, as part of the programme against hepatitis B, should help to control hepatitis C also.]

A multi-institutional, multinational collaborative training programme, focusing on research and training opportunities in the areas of HIV/AIDS, tuberculosis and emerging infections, for medical and scientific personnel from Poland and nine other countries of Central/Eastern Europe, has been established in New York State, funded by the Fogarty International Center of the National Institutes of Health. This programme has been developed to provide in-depth training for participants and to encourage the development of research programmes upon their return to their native countries (Morse and DeHovitz 2000). It is perhaps fortunate that tuberculosis has been included in the scope of this programme as, although the incidence has been declining steadily since 1994 (after an increase from 1989 to 1993), the fact that the new financing of the Polish healthcare system does not pay for contact tracing has led to concerns that some regions may actually be under reporting up to 40% of cases (Grzemska 2000).

National programme of rabies control

(Although of the six countries studied England and Malta are the only ones which are free of rabies in the animal population, the

subject is mentioned in this section because of its special significance.) The main reservoir of rabies in Poland is the red fox, the
virus having been established in that animal in the first decades of
the twentieth century by an adaptive process following a decline in
incidence among urban dogs and wolves. Other wild animals
affected include raccoons and, rather worryingly, bats (Bourhy *et
al.* 1999). Fifty years of mass dog vaccination has resulted in
considerable limitation of that epizootic, although the number of
rabid dogs indicates that the percentage of vaccinated dogs is still
too low in some districts. The problem of cat rabies depends on the
presence of dog and fox rabies; areas free of dog and fox rabies are
free of cat rabies.

Poland initiated mass oral vaccination of wild animals (by
inserting vaccine in bait) in 1993, initially along its western
border and subsequently gradually progressing to eastern districts
although some parts of the latter remain uncovered. Although
rabid foxes constitute approximately 70% of total animal infection,
they are responsible for only 9% of humans requiring to be vaccinated, usually as a result of indirect contact or licks; rabid dogs
and cats (mostly strays) are responsible for 75% of human vaccination, although they constitute only about 10% of total animal
infection. Until 2000, there had been no human rabies cases since
1986. This most recent case concerned a woman who was bitten
on the finger pulp by her own cat but did not seek vaccination.
Hence it is considered that more efficient health education
concerning the risk of rabies is required, alongside continuing
organisation of the vaccination of both domestic and wild animals
(Sadkowska-Todys 2001). [The oral immunisation of wildlife
animal reservoirs, aiming particularly at raccoons and skunks, is
currently being evaluated in the United States.]

Uganda

As mentioned in Chapter 3, the maximum delegation of responsibility to district level or below has been a marked feature of the
Health Sector Strategic Plan and this has had practical relevance
for the control of communicable diseases. Although the district is a
natural focus for this activity with its DDHS, District Government
Hospital and laboratory facilities, the fact that the ADDHS at
county level is almost certain to be the first *medical* person to be
made aware of any outbreak means that this individual may initially be the person best placed to respond by the implementation of

control measures. However, as was pointed out in Chapter 3, the flexibility in the roles of the DDHS *vis à vis* the ADDHSs of the constituent counties within the district is such that these doctors can work together as a team, particularly necessary if an outbreak covers more than one county. By the same token, if an outbreak affects more than one district then the flexibility extends further in that one of the ESD's epidemiologists can visit to assist with both investigation and control.

The National Disease Control Department currently operates six disease control programmes against:

- malaria
- HIV/AIDS
- vaccine-preventable diseases
- tuberculosis
- dracunculiasis (guinea worm disease)
- onchocerciasis (river blindness).

These programmes are largely funded by 'development partner donors' such as UNICEF, WHO, DFID, Danish International Development Assistance (DANIDA), etc. although there is also some Government financial support. Each of these programmes represents a composite 'package' of elements of not only *control* but also surveillance and prevention, thereby illustrating the interlocking nature of these activities (and also the occasional degree of artificiality in attempting to separate prevention from control, as concepts). The programmes were established before the ESD came into being and each had developed its own specific surveillance arrangements. When the ESD was created, it was concerned initially only with those communicable diseases not already covered by one of the six specific programmes, but it is currently responsible for a total overview of *all* disease surveillance, sharing relevant data with each of the individual programmes. This latter point is important as the donors continue to have an expectation that they can receive progress reports from the individual programme managers. These programmes have specific objectives and targets within the Health Sector Strategic Plan, for example, during the five-year period:

- to increase from 30% to 60% the proportion of the population that receive effective treatment for malaria within 24 hours of the onset of symptoms
- to attain a 25% reduction in HIV sero-prevalence

- to achieve 100% national coverage with community directly observed treatment system (DOTS) with regard to tuberculosis.

Of course, in general day-to-day events, a great deal of non-specific disease control is carried out at local level by the parish nurse and nursing assistant, working to agreed clinical guidelines, on the principle that if the problem settles down the matter can be considered closed. If it is felt that the matter cannot be handled locally, or if the condition appears to be one with epidemic potential (using the case definition approach described in Chapter 3), the problem can be very rapidly reported 'up-the-line' for appropriate investigation and public health intervention. The response to the recent outbreak of cholera in Hoima District, commencing in August 2002, illustrates this process very well. Additionally, a certain amount of illness is undoubtedly handled locally at village level by traditional practitioners, healers and herbalists. The role of such personnel is readily acknowledged and there is shortly to be a law introduced to coordinate and regulate their practice. Witchdoctors however are generally regarded as misguided, although in Rakai District in 1983/1984 there was a belief among some of the persons affected by what turned out to be AIDS that their symptoms were caused by witchcraft, so leading them to consult indigenous healers (Iliffe 1998).

One aspect of the control of communicable diseases in Uganda is so different from the situation in four of the other five countries examined in this study (France appears to occupy an intermediate position) that it requires a special brief mention. The concept of even the occasional need to use formal legal procedures to compel persons to comply with medical advice to avoid spreading infection is considered almost incomprehensible (Lamunu 2002). Ugandans generally feel very concerned, in a positive sense, about their state of health and therefore many greetings include enquiries about the health not only of the person being greeted but also of the person's family, relatives and friends, even of their domestic animals (Lubega 1997)! Even in the case of situations as serious as that of the 2002 Ebola epidemic, there is no recourse to the use of the law to restrict the movement of persons from one area to another. However, there *is* close monitoring of those who have been in contact with a suspected case for the possible development of the disease (Lwamafa 2002b).

CHAPTER 6

Reflections: what can be learned?

Historical events, especially those involving the movement of people – traders, explorers, colonisers, armies and more recently refugees – have unquestionably had a major impact on the incidence and pattern of communicable diseases. The mercantile prosperity of mediaeval Europe encouraged the movement, especially from the East, of those involved in trade; unfortunately the Black Death was frequently a fellow traveller. Furthermore, the Renaissance amounted to much more than a rebirth of learning in Europe; it also meant the dawn of an era of more extensive travel and exploration, associated with many fevers and plagues which nowadays would fall within the remit of the specialties of travel medicine or genitourinary medicine.

Many people, for example, believe that the arrival of syphilis in Europe can be linked to the return of Columbus's crew from the New World, a view supported by evidence of syphilitic changes in skulls found in North America, dating from before the arrival of Columbus. However, there is some contrary evidence in that there is a painting by Albrecht Dürer, dated 1484, eight years before Columbus's discovery, showing a man with lesions suggestive of syphilis. Perhaps understandably, American historians tend not to favour the former explanation; for example, George Rosen (1958), probably the greatest American public health historian, states 'Whatever its origin – *and this is not the place to discuss this problem* (my italics) – there is no question that the disease appeared in Europe in epidemic form at the close of the fifteenth century ...'. One might reasonably ask: 'Why not discuss it?' Certainly there was a degree of stigma about the condition right from the start. Rosen points out that the French called syphilis the 'Neapolitan disease' whereas the Italians referred to it as the 'Morbus Gallicus'. The English called it the 'French Pox' or the 'Great Pox', a literal translation of 'La Grosse Vérole', a reminder that in those days syphilis was an acute disease with high fever, fearful ulcers and a high mortality. Girolamo Fracastoro, a physician of Verona, added fuel to the flames when in 1530 he published a poem '*Syphilus sive morbus Gallicus*' (Syphilus or the French Disease). Syphilus was a young shepherd who, one might say, was unlucky in his choice of female companion. However, the poem did de-mystify the many theories surrounding the disease and the sexual nature of its spread became widely understood thereafter.

This tendency to link the origin of a new communicable disease (or even a new variant of a well-known one) with a particular country had, in fact, occurred even before the Renaissance was well under way. The year 1485 suggests to many people – and certainly to those who have seen Laurence Olivier's excellent film *Richard III* – the Battle of Bosworth Field. What appears to be less generally known is that, shortly after the battle, a communicable disease resembling severe influenza and referred to as 'the English Sweat' broke out among the victorious troops of Henry Tudor, spreading widely throughout the country, although not further afield, not even to Scotland! Perhaps it was the fact that it was such a violently acute illness with a brief period of communicability that limited its spread to a relatively short range; presumably those who did not die of the condition were too incapacitated to travel very far while they were still infectious. Subsequently we have encountered 'Spanish influenza', the deadly pandemic of 1918/1919 and more recently the 1957 'Asian flu' and in 1968 'Hong Kong flu' (referred to by some of the tabloids as 'Mao flu', making a link between the disease and the political administration in China, rather similar to the imagined link between typhus and bolshevism, referred to in Chapter 3). In earlier times the practice was no doubt a means of attributing blame, but more recently it has tended to indicate the location where the organism was first isolated and identified, for example *Salmonella Milwaukee*, thereby denoting an actual achievement. But even much earlier, the expression 'German measles' represented a tribute to workers in that country who, in the seventeenth century, had distinguished a condition which was almost certainly rubella from scarlet fever, rather than a xenophobic perception of a European neighbour!

Although, as mentioned in Chapter 3, brucellosis had probably been around in Malta in the sixteenth century under the name of 'erratic fever', it was only following the end of the Crimean War in 1856 that the disease assumed significant proportions, as a result of the garrisoning of British troops there. Colonisation could also contribute dramatically to disease incidence. In 1875, following

Britain's annexation of the Fiji Islands, the cruiser *Dido* arrived there with measles on board. The disease ran riot in such a non-immune community encountering the infection for the first time, killing 40 000 islanders – nearly a quarter of the population (McGrew 1985). The fact that Poland experienced centuries of wars with, and invasions by, neighbouring countries has had a profound influence on what might be termed its 'epidemiological experience'.

However, if we disregard, for the moment, Henry Ford's opinion that 'history is bunk', there are many versions of the contrary view, such as 'the only lesson that we learn from history is that mankind never learns from history' and 'he who cannot learn the lesson of history is destined to re-live it'. Certainly evidence supporting these latter expressions is not hard to find. Because of the breakdown of quarantine as a measure against the importation of cholera in 1831, England was very much in the vanguard of setting up a network of locally-based public health authorities. This, paradoxically, may have contributed to a relatively complacent attitude lasting well into the twentieth century, only to be dispelled by the emerging and re-emerging diseases of the 1970s and 1980s. On the other hand, some lessons of history can perhaps outlive their relevance. The total aversion to any element of compulsion with regard to routine childhood immunisation in England must certainly partly have its roots in accounts, passed down through the generations, of the violent opposition to smallpox vaccination resulting from the Government's overactive support for the procedure in the nineteenth century, making it first universally available, then free, and lastly compulsory.

The six countries studied display an interesting spectrum of attitudes towards the use of the law in both the prevention and control of communicable disease, ranging from having formidable powers on the Statute Book to a position which seems to indicate that the law has really no place in these matters. With regard to immunisation it should not be forgotten that, in addition to protecting the individual from developing a serious disease, the procedures help to protect the community by reducing the spread of infectious agents as a result of the development of herd immunity. Thus immunisation programmes must represent an attractive 'package' in the eyes of both governments and those responsible for promoting and managing public health activities. This is an important point to remember in any ethical debate on the question of compulsion. There is a broad similarity between the positions of the United States, France, Poland and Malta in that, unlike England or Uganda, all four formally require the carrying out of at least some of the routine childhood immunisation procedures.

However, within this broad similarity, there are subtle differences. On the face of it, the formality of the requirement appears to be most evident in Malta, with its reference to 'failure to comply with this duty ... the parent may be summoned by the Commissioner of Police ... the child may be immunised by Order of Court' and France, with its législation vaccinale by which 'a certain number of immunisations are rendered obligatory by texts of law'. Of course to understand the French attitude to compulsory immunisation one has to try to understand the culture of the country, especially in relation to obeying the law. Michel Rey (1980) has perhaps offered the most useful insight when, as mentioned in Chapter 4, he includes France as one of 'les pays du Sud, de culture méditerranéenne, de tendance légaliste par tradition latine, s'appuyant sur les lois, mais assez laxiste dans l'application de celles-ci' (... the countries of the South, with a Mediterranean culture, of a legalistic inclination by latin tradition, relying on laws, but being sufficiently latitudinarian with regard to their application). Referring to France specifically, he states 'Elle reflète la tradition "latine": législation très développée, mais appliquée sans grande rigeur, conformément au tempérament national individualiste. Elle s'insère dans un système sanitaire qui ne manque pas de paradoxes'. (It reflects the 'latin' tradition: well-developed legislation, but not applied with any great strictness, in accordance with a national individualistic disposition. It fits it into a health system which does not lack paradoxes.)

The Polish approach is particularly interesting in that the procedures are 'obowiązkowe', i.e. obligatory, but not 'przymusowe', i.e. compulsory. These two terms require a degree of explanation. The former implies a duty or obligation and therefore in this context means that every child is obliged to be immunised; nevertheless the final decision remains with the individual, in this instance the parent. The latter, implying as it does compulsion *by force if necessary* represents a concept totally unacceptable to Poles whose spirit rebels against such ideas in relation to childhood immunisation (and, for that matter, to many other social issues). How then is routine childhood immunisation achieved? Quite simply, Polish people are very mindful of their history and the part that epidemics have played in it, and have a good understanding of the role of vaccination and immunisation in containing and controlling these epidemics. As a result, Poles have a strong belief in the efficacy of such measures and anti-vaccination movements are not popular in their country. Furthermore, there is a considerable measure of community support for the idea of herd immunity and anyone trying to avoid immunisation comes under considerable pressure from other members of the family, from friends and from neighbours. Hence the concept of 'obligation to society' is by itself sufficient to ensure individual and community protection (Magdzik 2002a).

Perhaps the most indirect approach to compulsion is to be found in the United States where evidence of immunisation has to be produced before any child is allowed to enter kindergarten, school or any other child group facility. Using the local schools and other child-care centres as 'enforcing agencies' on behalf of the State Department of Health does appear to be a useful way of securing that non-immunised children are not allowed to put others at risk. However, for quite a separate reason, not being allowed to attend school on that account may well seem ethically questionable in certain communities with low educational level of parents, low socio-economic status, large family size, young parental age and non-white race or ethnicity where, as pointed out in Chapter 4, take-up rates tend to be low. This could, in fact, be seen as a kind of 'double whammy' for the affected children – missing out on both immunisation *and* education. It would be interesting to know to what extent the federal means-tested food voucher system for needy infants and young children, referred to in Chapter 4, might really make a major impact on those twin disadvantages. Certainly such research as has been carried out is encouraging; immunisation levels have been reported to be increased by 36–40% in children enrolled in these programmes (Hutchins and Rosenthal 1994).

The absence of compulsion in this field is also worthy of study. England's history may well be unique in going from one extreme to the other. The Government's initial active support for smallpox vaccination in the nineteenth century, especially the compulsory element, soon had to be modified in the light of the public disquiet and the consequent continued evasion of the vaccination laws by parents. The term 'disquiet' may well be considered somewhat of an understatement when one considers the summoning and jailing of parents, the public demonstrations and the riots! However, it is interesting to note that, in the wake of these events, there was no overt 'U-turn' on the part of the Government of the day, or of any subsequent one for that matter, on the question of compulsion. The concept of conscientious objection no doubt satisfied both sides (neither the author nor his father, for example, were vaccinated as infants, 'advantage' having been taken of this let-out clause), until the 1946 NHS Act wrapped up the whole matter rather neatly by making no reference to compulsion with regard to any aspect of vaccination or immunisation. [As a side-issue, the author has found during over 30 years of public health practice that the term 'vaccination' in relation to any routine childhood immunisation procedure may tend to worry some parents; the word 'immunisation' does not generally appear to have this effect, although this may now be changing because of the way in which the media have handled the MMR situation.]

In these circumstances it would appear reasonable to speculate that the history of smallpox vaccination in England is the principal reason for routine childhood immunisation being totally free from compulsion, direct or indirect, and dependent only on information-giving, education, encouragement, persuasion and good organisation within primary care. This includes, more recently, financial incentives for general practitioners to reach specific coverage targets. However, there may well be a further factor operating which could be influencing the English attitude. Michel Rey (1980), in contrasting England with France, says of the former that it is one of 'les pays du Nord, Anglo-Saxon, socio-démocrate, de tradition libérale et pragmatique, n'imposant pas d'obligation légale, admettant éventuellement l'objection de conscience, faisant largement appel à l'éducation sanitaire, non sans recourir aussi à diverses contraintes administratives et psychologiques' (... the countries of the North, Anglo-Saxon, social democratic, with a liberal and pragmatic tradition, not imposing legal obligations, possibly allowing objection on grounds of conscience, broadly appealing to health education, but also not without resorting to administrative and psychological constraints).

In practice, the methods of calculating immunisation coverage in England, the United States, France and Uganda differ so greatly that precise comparisons cannot reasonably be made. However, in Malta and Poland, the evaluation processes appear to be as rigid as the requirement for immunisation itself, and therefore limited comparisons with England would appear to be worthwhile. On this basis, the lack of legal enforcement in England does not appear to be a cause of poor performance in this aspect of disease prevention (with the comparatively recent exception of protection against measles, mumps and rubella, for the reasons outlined in Chapter 4).

It is perhaps tempting to come to the conclusion that the English experience shows that, generally speaking, compulsion is not necessary for successful coverage of routine childhood immunisation and that the Americans, French, Poles and Maltese could dispense with it. However, this makes enormous assumptions about the 'portability' of systems from one country to another and it is important to speculate why the informal approach has been successful in England. Firstly, the NHS has set routine childhood immunisation firmly within general practice with strong financial incentives. Secondly, the computerised system operated by the PCTs guarantees the outward and inward flow of the relevant forms by the local general practitioners. Thirdly, the Department of Health has from 1963 regularly issued its publication *Immunisation against Infectious Disease* which is used by all healthcare personnel as an authoritative source of up-to-date information. Lastly, health education on this topic and a willingness to answer questions, by midwives and health visitors, begin in pregnancy and form a core element of any discussions with parents soon after the birth.

The sheer size and diversity of the United States, along with the combination of both private and public sector provision and the absence of a national health service to coordinate and facilitate the arrangements, would probably render an effective programme unmanageable, not to mention the likely opposition of many parents who would probably see such a change as putting *their* children at risk. This last point would almost certainly apply very strongly in Poland also, for the reasons given above. In both France and Malta, such a shift in policy would run counter to what has been traditionally accepted and might well result in a decrease in coverage because of misunderstanding. 'If the government no longer *requires* us to do this, it's probably not really necessary after all!' might be one reaction (Agius Muscat 1998). After all, in France the formal requirement to be vaccinated against smallpox was discontinued following global eradication of the disease, and against typhoid fever when improvement in living standards greatly reduced the risk. It will be interesting to observe whether Uganda will be able to sustain its informal approach and at the same time achieve its coverage targets or whether, as some speculate, a USA-style arrangement may be called for by which children will have to demonstrate proof of protection against at least some of the diseases before being allowed to start school.

More generally, there could be situations in which, for example, a developing nation with insufficient resources devoted to healthcare, and possibly literacy problems, might feel that it has to adopt a firmer approach to securing adequate coverage in the short term. A similar situation may exist during hostilities, with significant movement of refugees, as was illustrated by the UNICEF immunisation programmes for Kosovar children in Albania, Macedonia and Montenegro. In the long term, of course, it is hoped that education will lead to a situation in which parents feel that protection by immunisation is their child's *right*, rather than something which their governments impose upon them by law.

Returning to the situation in England, mention was made in Chapter 4 of what an editorial in the *BMJ* had referred to as 'the discomfort of patient power' in situations in which patients may choose to disregard their doctors' advice and do something which their doctors regard as odd, even crazy. The editorial concluded that doctors would have to live with 'irrational' decisions by the public. This phenomenon is currently a live issue with regard to the (negative) reaction of a small proportion of parents to the question of MMR immunisation. This is illustrated by the overall decline in coverage from 92% to 84% between 1995/96 and 2001/2002 (with consequent measles outbreaks in those parts of the country with the lowest coverage) in spite of the extensive research findings showing no link between the procedure and autism. It raises some thought-provoking philosophical questions. For example, if all the evidence from research throughout the world had incriminated MMR as having significant risks but Dr Wakefield as a single individual asserted that it was safe, would most parents accept his views and act accordingly? Certainly not, but where therefore is the logic of accepting a lone viewpoint against the findings of the world research community? Clearly this is not simply a matter of logic.

Philosophy apart, this situation presents post-modern England with a novel kind of public health problem for which there is no obvious solution. Given the country's culture and traditions, compulsion is clearly out of the question, even the 'indirect' compulsion witnessed in the United States; i.e. it would be difficult to use maintained schools as 'enforcing agencies', although private schools could no doubt decide this matter for themselves. Therefore, as parents represent the sole arbiters, it is doubly important that they have access to all the relevant facts to allow them to make an informed decision. This information should, of course, include a reminder of the wretchedness of the experience of suffering from the actual disease (an early poster had the caption **Measles is Misery**), and its potential for complications such as middle ear infection, pneumonia and neurological damage, alongside the wealth of research evidence concerning the safety of the vaccine.

Another factor may turn out to be the reaction of other parents, i.e how they may feel if *their* children are put at risk as a result of infection being introduced into any group by a non-immunised child. There is already some anecdotal evidence that some playgroups and nursery schools are quietly declining to take children who have not been immunised, a state of affairs that would be applauded by the great majority of parents in the United States; in Poland, it would be regarded as the only sensible course of action. Why the differences in approach? Is it because being ill in the United States can be costly as well as unpleasant? Is it simply that Poland's past vulnerability to communicable diseases has instilled into the population an unusually strong tradition of appreciating the value of protective vaccines?

The 1988 Acheson Committee report *Public Health in England* agreed a definition of its subject matter as 'the science and art of preventing disease, prolonging life and promoting health *through organised efforts of society*' (my italics). This concept is interesting in that it makes it clear that the issues go far beyond the actions of public health professionals, although the frustrations of the latter can readily be understood against a background – almost a mantra – of 'if preventable, why not prevented?'. Simply standing back and placing the responsibility totally upon parents may seem to the doctor rather like opting out but if, as mentioned in Chapter 4, excessive reassurance proves counterproductive, giving factual information and being prepared to answer all questions may be as far as one can go. [However, it may possibly be worthwhile looking at the experience of other European countries, such as Sweden, Ireland and Austria, which also have no formal requirements for routine childhood immunisation.]

There is, of course, also the matter of being completely honest about the understandable wish of the Government to achieve a high level of herd immunity, an issue which overlaps with, but is not quite the same as, the protection of the individual child – presumably the prime motivation of any parent. Middle class 'table-talk' may well create the impression that, in such matters, trust in the medical profession has declined a little. However, as was recently pointed out in a Reith Lecture, actions do not necessarily match words; general practitioner surgeries are as busy as ever, and the annual MORI poll of the most trusted professionals or occupational groups, carried out in February 2003, placed doctors, just after nurses, at the top.

Although, as mentioned in Chapter 5, most people cooperate well when requested to take measures to prevent the spread of infection, recourse to legal powers is rarely needed to ensure that others are not put at risk. The fact that the law so rarely *has* to be used should not conceal the possibility that the very knowledge of its existence may well contribute to informal compliance. [For example, when the author was a practising public health physician in Coventry, in situations in which he was obliged to request some action regarded by the recipient as unwelcome or a great nuisance, he was not infrequently asked: 'Could I be made to?' On having the legal position fully explained, the majority tended to cooperate informally, even though sometimes somewhat reluctantly.]

In this sphere, there appears to be a broad similarity between the approaches of England, the United States, Poland and Malta in that in all four countries the relevant public health physician has legal powers which can be utilised, if necessary, to require a person *inter alia* to submit to medical examination, to be excluded from work, or to be admitted to hospital and detained there. Chapter 5 showed that France, by comparison, with its apparent aversion to the restriction of liberty, seems to cope with these problems without the back-up of any legal compulsion, apart from dire situations such as major epidemics, and in Uganda the idea that the law would need to be used at all, for such common-sense actions, is apparently incomprehensible.

The situation in England is somewhat paradoxical. From the middle of the nineteenth century the country was well in the vanguard of creating a locally-based, medically-led public health service with appropriate powers. However, by 1988, when two public inquiries had made it necessary for there to be a complete reappraisal of the public health function, the law on the control of communicable disease was perceived as very dated, appearing to be still largely based on nineteenth century concepts. Although this reappraisal called for a complete review of the relevant law, this has not yet taken place nor does there seem to be much general discussion of the topic. The coming into being of the proposed Health Protection Agency in April 2003 may provide a fresh opportunity for progress to be made.

If England is sometimes perceived as insular, not only geographically but also culturally, Poland perhaps presents the most dramatic contrast. In Chapter 3, reference was made to its having been described as the most easterly country in western Europe, and therefore in the path of the frequent westward spread of such diseases as plague, cholera, typhus and influenza (and, more recently, multidrug-resistant tuberculosis). Being *in medias res*, so to speak, to such an extent has certainly governed the country's attitude to communicable diseases. This has been mentioned in Chapter 4 in relation to routine childhood immunisation, but it is also reflected in both the firmness of the legal authority given to the dyrektor of the local sanepid who can, if need be, call upon the police or City Guard to enforce control activities, and the responsiveness of the public which tends to render such enforcement unnecessary. Certainly Polish people appear to be acutely conscious of the potential menace of communicable diseases and readily see the wisdom of protecting their health and that of their families and the wider community.

In the United States there appears currently to be a very active debate on the various aspects of the subject, not only because of the post-September 11 2001 situation but also because of an ongoing need to clarify the respective roles of the individual states and the federal government, against a background of wider discussion of what Gostin (1986) has referred to as the classic problem for public health jurisprudence, namely the tension between protection of the public health and protection of civil liberties, more specifically, in this instance, the extent to which the state may restrain its citizens in order to interrupt the spread of communicable disease. Because of this, it is perhaps worthwhile briefly examining some of this thinking as some of the ideas may justify discussion in other countries.

Gostin's initial argument is that public health laws are based on an antiquated conception of communicable disease control which does not take into account advances in scientific knowledge. He considers, for example, that most of these laws were written when sciences such as epidemiology were in their infancy and that consequently concepts such as isolation and quarantine have been founded on an incomplete understanding of the means of spread of infection. He also contends that what he refers to as the concept of 'public health necessity' lacks proper criteria for making important public health decisions and that consequently the balance between public protection and individual rights is left to the discretion of public health officials. He argues strongly for these criteria to be based on contemporary knowledge of the mechanisms of disease spread and that, as the exercise of compulsory powers may be counterproductive, a graded series of less restrictive powers, for example based on education and counselling within a 'community health order', should be available to the public health authority. One of his main criticisms of public health practice is that it is based on the assumption that it is better that any risk of error in the management of a situation be on the side of a more cautious (i.e. restrictive) approach. However, some public health physicians might have certain reservations about his 'less restrictive community-based powers' and might yet have to be convinced that it would be a straightforward matter to make a clear distinction between safe and unsafe behaviours while participating in social activities.

Nevertheless, even firmer measures for the control of certain diseases *have* also represented a feature of the United States' scene. For example, in 1993 the New York City Department of Health, alarmed at the rapid increase in the incidence of tuberculosis, amended its Health Code to permit compulsory actions to protect the public health. The amendment allowed the Commissioner of Health to order compulsory directly observed therapy and, as a last resort, civil detention of persistently non-compliant patients until completion of treatment. A study of patients dealt with in this way between September 1993 and September 1994 showed that only 15% of non-compliant patients needed to be detained and that civil detention proved effective in these cases by ensuring the completion of treatment (Feldman *et al.* 1997). A further study, covering patients from April 1993 to April 1995, confirmed that for most, even those with severe social problems, completion of treatment could usually be achieved without compulsion and that the less restrictive measure of mandatory directly observed therapy was often effective. Detention was used only when patients posed a serious threat to public health but, when applied, it was highly successful in ensuring complete treatment (Gasner *et al.* 1999).

As Annas (2002) has pointed out, post-September 11 2001, the public health climate in the United States has changed. Concern over the looming threat of bioterrorism had been evident for some time; Henderson (1999) was arguing strongly for a strengthening of the public health infrastructure and in the following year CDC Atlanta produced its 'Strategic Plan for Preparedness and Response', including the public health powers which it envisaged as necessary in a bioterrorism event. Annas explains how the anthrax attacks through the US mail confronted local, state and federal public health officials with the prospect of having to deal with a real bioterrorist attack. As the latter represents both a state and a federal crime, the Federal Bureau of Investigation (FBI) and CDC Atlanta took the lead, on that occasion, in investigating all the anthrax mail attacks, and CDC released its proposed Model State Emergency Health Powers Act on 23 October 2001. This gave the state governor and public health officials very wide-ranging authority over physicians, citizens and healthcare facilities in the state. Criticisms of the Model Act, based on views that its provisions were too draconian, led to a revised version being released on 21 December 2001 as a 'draft for discussion' but Annas expresses the view that the suggested powers to be given to officials are still excessive and that some of the concepts, for example quarantine, are arbitrary. Clearly the tension between protection of the public health and protection of civil liberties is going to continue to be a subject of considerable concern, perhaps far beyond the United States.

A 'culture' of frequent major reorganisations of the services which are concerned *inter alia* with the control of communicable diseases has certainly been a prominent feature of the English scene – four since 1974. The first of these had as its main thrust the integration of local hospital and community services so that, theoretically at least, all the different kinds of care and treatment that an individual might need should be readily available from an integrated health service. Unfortunately, when the integrated service came into being, communicable disease control had apparently become a casualty of the more compelling discussions over health service unification, and new relationships with local government. In particular the abolition of the post of Medical Officer of Health, with its statutory requirement for the additional qualification to ensure professional competence in the discharge of the duties, represented to many a premature dismantling of a system geared to health protection. The 1982 're-structuring' simply represented a rationalisation of general health service provision and it was not until six years later that the Acheson Report, in the wake of the Stanley Royd and Stafford outbreaks, once more brought communicable disease control centre stage, suggesting what was thought at the time to be the definitive solution. The most recent attempt, namely the proposed inclusion of this area of work in the responsibilities of the new Health Protection Agency, remains to be evaluated in due course.

Thus during a period of less than 30 years the responsibilities will have been exercised consecutively by the Medical Officer of Health, the Medical Officer for Environmental Health, the Consultant in Communicable Disease Control and now the relevant employee of the Health Protection Agency, the expertise required being first generic, then specialised and finally once more generic, while accountability will have passed from local government, via the NHS, to a (presumed) non-governmental organisation, and lastly back to the NHS as a Special Health Authority (SHA). The uncertainties arising from such frequent and fundamental changes cannot in any way contribute to the notion of a clearly defined career path for anyone interested in this kind of work and anecdotal evidence would tend to bear this out.

The other five countries do not appear to have been obsessed during this period with the need for such radical reorganisation in this field. Admittedly France has seen two structural changes in the responsibility for national surveillance, from the Direction Générale de la Santé to the Réseau National de Santé Publique and subsequently to the Institut de Veille Sanitaire, but the responsible public health physician at local level has remained the well-established Médecin Inspecteur de Santé Publique. Similarly in the United States, Poland, Malta and Uganda, such minor changes as have occurred have tended to represent consolidation of existing arrangements associated with acquiring the benefits of scientific discoveries and the introduction of developing applications of information technology.

Disregarding the familiar political rhetoric by which many governments tend to laud the merits of decentralisation and/or delegation, and pledge to implement them, this dimension *does* actually have a bearing on some aspects of the subject matter of this study. One interesting illustration of this can be found in contrasting the extent and nature of professional autonomy in communicable disease control at local level afforded to the CCDC in England *vis-à-vis* the MISP in France.

The CCDC, after at least four years of specialist (i.e. non-generic) training, must clear the formidable hurdle of the Advisory Appointments Committee but, if successful, is deemed to be competent to exercise his or her professional judgement in handling local outbreaks, reporting to or seeking guidance from 'above' in only a limited number of (unusual) situations. The MISP's training, on the other hand, as was detailed in Chapter 5, covers an extremely wide range of public health topics among which communicable disease control represents only a limited area of study. Hence it is totally reasonable and sensible for the incumbent to look to 'the centre' for detailed guidance, whether this is from the relevant circulars which have been issued by Central Government or more personally from the medical epidemiologists of the Institut de Veille Sanitaire in Paris. This approach can be seen as characteristically French in terms of tradition. For example, a circular of 2 May 1805 from the Minister of the Interior to the prefect of each département instructed them in the proper procedures for handling epidemics, specified that an 'epidemic doctor' be named in each arrondissement and spelled out the status and duties of these doctors (Ackerman 1990). Péquignot (1954), in a paper on health administration, illustrated the policy perfectly when he stated 'Since the method of dealing with questions of techniques in preventive work is essentially by means of national circulars, it is difficult to imagine a policy of official services different in the Savoy and in the Morbihan'. Brockington (1967), commenting on this, expressed the view that in England it would be difficult to imagine them the same! This difference in philosophical viewpoint is evident in the law itself. As Cairns and McKeon (1995) have pointed out, the French approach is essentially deductive, starting from broad principles which are then applied to individual cases, whereas the British approach is basically empirical, believing that all knowledge is derived from experience and that broad principles can only be developed on the basis of observation.

Malta's small size and 'compact' medical community – one main state general hospital, one medical school and one medical association – have clearly made centralisation not only inevitable but sensible. The arrangement by which the three MOHs work in the same central office in Valletta, along with the principal medical officer responsible for disease surveillance, and sharing the same computer hardware, not only promotes coordination and team-working but also provides an optimal model of the close integration of surveillance and control activities advocated in Chapter 2, a convincing illustration of 'small is beautiful'. Another benefit of the closely-knit medical community in which individuals are known to one another is that lines of communication are short and opportunities abound for collaborative ventures between epidemiologists and clinicians. An excellent example, briefly mentioned in Chapter 3, is represented by the exploration of the possibilities of establishing 'sentinel' surveillance, based on the French model, by creating an electronic link between general practitioners and the Disease Surveillance Branch of the Department of Public Health so that the doctors could notify cases by e-mail.

Conversely, the sheer size of the United States and the question of 'states' rights' together mean that, apart from the limited federal role in this field, the concept of decentralisation is irrelevant. The process really works in reverse as, according to the Constitution, any powers *not* given to the federal government remain with the states. Against this background, it says a great deal for the Council of State and Territorial Epidemiologists' capacity to reach professional consensus on key public health issues affecting an enormous total population living in widely differing climates and terrains.

Decentralisation, along with maximum delegation of responsibility and authority, are also marked features of Uganda's Health Sector Strategic Plan and consequently have had a major impact on the arrangements for the prevention and control of communicable diseases. Originally this was just as far as district level, as this is a 'natural' unit for these purposes (especially the organisation of immunisation services), but more recently the extension of the process to the county level has perhaps given the latter a clearer sense of identity in healthcare terms. However, one can see strong arguments for disease *surveillance* being retained centrally in the Epidemiological Surveillance Division in Kampala, to allow the overall picture to be viewed and also to provide the relevant data for planning, with the proviso that collated information is fed back 'down the line' to keep the data providers motivated. In all these respects modern Uganda can be regarded as fortunate in that, unlike the other five countries in this study, it is a relatively new country, not only following independence but also re-emerging vigorously following civil conflict, and is therefore well placed to take a cool look at its future health needs and plan accordingly.

Although in Chapter 2, Figure 2.4 (*see* p 21) attempts to demonstrate a logical line of demarcation between control and prevention, the topic of condoms in relation to sexually-transmitted infections illustrates the conceptual difficulty of maintaining this line too rigidly. Why, for example, apart from the purpose of contraception, do people wear male or female condoms? Is it to protect themselves or their partners (perhaps at the partner's insistence)? The views of the American Public Health Association on this matter are set out as follows:

> 'The only sure way to avoid infection through sex is to abstain from sexual intercourse or to engage in mutually monogamous sexual intercourse with someone known to be uninfected. In other situations, latex condoms must be used correctly every time a person has vaginal, anal or oral sex' (APHA 2000).

Of the six countries studied, Malta with its population 98% Roman Catholic is the one in particular which has had to find ways of reconciling religious observance with health protection. For those who are able to accept 'chastity before marriage and faithfulness within it', there are presumably no problems. For others, there are the condom-dispensing machines in night-clubs, etc. Although Poland also has a majority Roman Catholic population, anecdotal evidence suggests that, generally, people tend to make up their own minds about such personal matters and Polish-produced condoms (prezerwatywa) are available from most kiosks and from some pharmacists.

In the fight against STIs, it is important to recognise that countries can vary greatly in the extent to which it may be possible to discuss sexual matters openly. Chapter 4 makes it clear that, of the six countries studied, Malta is the most reticent and Uganda the least inhibited. In fact, in the latter country the sexual aspects of human relationships regularly feature quite strongly in the Press, often in articles written in a light-hearted and entertaining manner, for example a full page item headed 'Can women ejaculate, or is it just peeing?' (*The Monitor* 30 August 2002). In such a relaxed climate of opinion, it becomes quite a straightforward matter to have news items dealing with, for example, 90 000 male condoms and 110 female condoms being given out free in five districts (*New Vision* 26 November 2002) and the Government's plan to import 120 million condoms (*New Vision* 15 February 2003). Furthermore President Museveni, on opening the Thirty-sixth Commonwealth Regional Health Ministers' Conference, stated that he had issued a directive to the effect that every headteacher must convene a school general assembly every two weeks to address the students on the subject of HIV/AIDS (*New Vision* 19 November 2002).

However, in any country, economic factors may also be relevant; for example, as Alcabes (2000) has emphasised, in situations where women without marketable skills are forced into providing sexual services to support their children, their lack of empowerment makes it unlikely that they will be in a position to insist on a condom being used.

Although a book of this kind might, theoretically at least, allow the drawing of conclusions from the findings as a basis for defining a model of good practice, the author makes no such claim as, in such a limited and semi-anecdotal study, this would be over-ambitious. In any event, it is hoped that what has been shown is that no single model could be imposed for general application. However, a number of issues appear to be worthy of some consideration.

In the developed world, one normally thinks of the process of surveillance as beginning with a notification by a clinician or a report from a microbiologist. Laboratory-based reporting is particularly well developed in the United States, for example, and England is moving in that direction as part of the strategy of the Communicable Disease Surveillance Centre. However, it would be a pity if, as a consequence of this, less attention were to be paid to notifications by clinicians which can often allow an earlier public health control response. It has to be accepted that securing the latter very much depends on two things. Firstly, clinicians need to regard notification as a high priority activity on their part, i.e. they require strong motivation; secondly, they need to receive sufficient feedback to *remain* motivated. It is hoped that some of the examples given show where careful thought has resulted in successful responses. The introduction of the 'sentinel' notification system in France in the 1980s is particularly worthy of note. Also, by taking the trouble to find out which factors are relevant to motivation, Chauvin and Valleron (1995) have shown that general practitioners can clearly distinguish between notification for urgent public health control measures and that for longer-term surveillance, and with regard to the latter they are particularly interested in uncommon and serious diseases and those which are readily preventable. Certainly it would seem worthwhile for the district public health physician, in any country, to take the initiative in contacting general practitioners, initially through their local representative machinery, to explore the advantages of this kind of partnership (hence the author's plea, in Chapter 3, that no surveillance system should be regarded as *passive*!).

A willingness, or otherwise, to learn from the experience of other countries has almost certainly had relevance to the development of surveillance systems. One could argue that England could have had an effective system from the late 1950s, modelled on that of the United States; both could have gleaned much from Poland's actions following the First World War. Malta and Uganda clearly did not try to re-invent the wheel and very sensibly drew upon existing templates prepared by CDC Atlanta and WHO Geneva.

In the developing world laboratory facilities are less likely to be readily available. Uganda's approach, depending largely on agreed clinical case definitions (fine-tuned to the needs of a variety of individuals with different levels of knowledge), demonstrates how a notification system can begin to operate from the periphery well in advance of the involvement of any medical practitioner, with the messages moving towards the centre through a hierarchy of expertise. Although, as this last example shows, approaches to surveillance have to take into account a variety of circumstances applying to the particular country, what emerges is a shared concept which is essentially *professional*, with considerable enthusiasm for networking, and which, unlike preventive and control measures, does not come with any cultural 'baggage' such as legal requirements or penalties!

What of the future?

As communicable diseases have always been with us, one must assume that they will continue to represent hazards to humans. The primary aim of all species is to survive; pathogenic microbes are no exception and, with their adaptability in acquiring human hosts as a base for multiplication and spread, they seem well suited to survival. Considerable unevenness of social concern about communicable diseases has been evident thoughout recorded history. Positive action has tended to be sporadic, mainly as a result of a government becoming acutely anxious over a perceived imminent danger; lack of such threats has tended to result in a degree of complacency until the next cause for alarm. Population movement between countries – economic migration, asylum-seeking, religious pilgrimages, or simply business or holiday travel (including 'sex tourism') – will continue to favour microbial spread. SARS is the most recent communicable disease to give cause for alarm and it is impossible at the present time to forecast the course of this epidemic.

Similarly, at the time of writing it is particularly difficult to predict the possible impact of bioterrorism. It may surprise some to know that the threat of this kind of attack is not a recent development; when the author was doing his National Service in the Royal Army Medical Corps in the 1950s, the basic training included an overview of what was referred to as ABC (atomic, bacteriological and chemical) warfare. Particularly in the United States, much work has been published on the topic since the end of the Second World War, with increasingly loud demands for a strengthening of the public health infrastructure which would play a key role in any episode of this kind. However, this issue needs to be considered against the overall global burden of communicable disease prevalence; even without this specific threat, one should never regard such diseases as 'virtually eliminated as health problems'.

Notifiable diseases in England

Under the Public Health (Control of Disease) Act (1984)

Cholera
Plague
Relapsing fever

Smallpox
Typhus

Under the Public Health (Infectious Diseases) Regulations (1988)

Acute encephalitis
Acute poliomyelitis
Anthrax
Diphtheria
Dysentery (amoebic or bacillary)
Leprosy
Leptospirosis
Malaria
Measles
Meningitis
Meningococcal septicaemia
(without meningitis)
Mumps

Ophthalmia neonatorum
Paratyphoid fever
Rabies
Rubella
Scarlet fever
Tetanus
Tuberculosis
Typhoid fever
Viral haemorrhagic fever
Viral hepatitis
Whooping cough
Yellow fever

Food poisoning is separately notifiable under food hygiene legislation.

Future arrangements for surveillance in England

The arrangements for communicable disease surveillance in England are about to change as a result of radical restructuring. The Government's 2002 report *Getting Ahead of the Curve: a strategy for combatting infectious diseases (including other aspects of health protection)* declared the intention of creating a new National Infection Control and Health Protection Agency – subsequently referred to as simply the Health Protection Agency (HPA) – in order to provide a more integrated approach to *all* aspects of health protection including chemical and radiological hazards. The HPA is therefore due to absorb the existing functions of the PHLS (including its Communicable Disease Surveillance Centre), the Centre for Applied Microbiological Research, the National Radiological Protection Board and the National Focus for Chemical Incidents.

The HPA is due to be operational by April 2003 but it will only be established as an executive non-departmental public body by April 2004. CCDCs are to have their contracts transferred from PCTs to the Agency on 1 April 2003 and they are likely to be grouped into local units covering the territory of two or more PCTs.

At the time of writing (February 2003), details of how the HPA will operate are still being finalised, according to the Department of Health.

Reportable diseases in Oklahoma

AIDS	Leptospirosis
Amebiasis	Lyme disease
Anthrax	Malaria
Botulism	**Measles (rubeola)**
Brucellosis	**Meningococcal infection**
Campylobacter infection	Mumps
Chlamydia	**Pertussis**
Cholera	**Plague**
Congenital rubella syndrome	Poliomyelitis
Diphtheria	**Rabies** (Human)
Encephalitis	Reye syndrome
Giardiasis	Rocky Mountain spotted
Gonorrhoea	fever
Haemophilus influenzae **invasive disease**	Rubella
	Salmonella infection
Hepatitis A	*Shigella* infection
Hepatitis B	Syphilis
Hepatitis non-A, non-B (includes hepatitis C)	Tetanus
	Toxic shock syndrome
Hepatitis, unspecified	Tuberculosis
HIV infection	Tularaemia
Kawasaki disease	**Typhoid fever**
Legionnaires' disease	Yellow fever

Diseases shown in **bold** need to be reported promptly by telephone

SARS: An important lesson?

WHO has pointed out (Communicable Disease Surveillance and Response Update 83) that 19 June 2003 marked the hundredth day since it first alerted the world, on 12 March, to the SARS threat. As mentioned in Chapter 1, by the end of June globally there had been around 8500 cases with over 800 deaths. But the WHO report also stated that during June the number of new cases had gradually dwindled to a daily handful, and concluded that the global outbreak was clearly coming under control.

Chapter 1 drew attention to population movements, especially air travel, as a key human factor contributing to the appearance and spread of new infections. SARS probably illustrates this phenomenon more clearly than any other disease mentioned in that chapter. Its brief section entitled 'How are the various authorities responding?' was written before the outbreak had come to public attention. Accordingly, it is salutary to re-read it with SARS in mind, especially the references to declaring the prevention of infectious diseases to be a high priority, to improving surveillance, to planning an increase in services for control and to the need for international co-operation, including the particular importance of the Global Outbreak and Response Network which WHO has operated since April 2000.

On a rather parochial note, it is gratifying to observe that, within the UK, the surveillance and control arrangements were such that the four probable cases were quickly identified, admitted to hospital and discharged in good health without any secondary cases occuring.

References

Ackerman EB (1990) *Health Care in the Parisian Countryside, 1800–1914*. Rutgers University Press, New Brunswick and London.

Agius Muscat H (1998) Personal communication. Interview with author, 25 November, Department of Health Information, Gwardamangia, Malta.

Alcabes P (2000) *New Epidemics and Society in Transition: AIDS in Poland and Eastern Europe*. Oral presentation at International Conference on Emerging, Re-emerging and Drug-Resistant Infections in Central and Eastern Europe on 28 March 2000 at the National Institute of Hygiene, Warsaw.

Allwright SPA (1988) Whooping cough. In AJ Silman and SPA Allwright (eds) *Elimination and Reduction of Diseases*. Oxford University Press, Oxford.

Altekruse SF, Stern NJ, Fields PI and Swerdlow DL (1999) Campylobacter jejuni – an emerging foodborne pathogen. *Emerging Infectious Diseases*. **5**: 28.

Alter MJ, Kruszon-Morgan D, Nainan OV *et al.* (1999) The prevalence of hepatitis C virus infection in the United States, 1988 through 1994. *New England Journal of Medicine*. **341**: 556–62.

Amato-Gauci AJ (2002) Personal communication. E-mail to author 17 July.

American Public Health Association (APHA) (1995) *Control of Communicable Diseases Manual* (16e). AS Benenson (ed.). APHA, Washington DC.

American Public Health Association (APHA) (2000) *Control of Communicable Diseases Manual* (17e). J Chinn (ed.). APHA, Washington DC.

Annas, GJ (2002) Bioterrorism, public health, and civil liberties. *New England Journal of Medicine*. **346**: 1337–41.

Bahá'í International Community (1999) In Uganda, community health workers effect long term changes. *One Country* (online newsletter). **11**: Issue 2, July–September.

Balińska MA (1995) Assistance and not mere relief: the Epidemic Commission of the League of Nations. In: PJ Weindling (ed.) *International Health Organisations and Movements 1918–1939*. Cambridge University Press, Cambridge.

Balińska MA (1998) *For the Good of Humanity*. Central European University Press, Budapest.

Balińska MA (2000) Report and commentary on the Conference on Emerging, Re-emerging and Drug-Resistant Infections in Central and Eastern Europe, Warsaw, March 28–29. Direction Générale de la Santé, Paris.

Balińska MA (2001) At the Crossroads of European Public Health: the case of Poland. (Unpublished).

Bardhan M (1999) Personal communication. Telephone conversation with author, 9 April.

Begg NT, Gill ON and White JM (1989) COVER (Cover of Vaccination Evaluated Rapidly): description of the England and Wales scheme. *Public Health.* **103**: 81–9.

Benagiano G, Rezza G and Vella S (2000) Condom use for preventing the spread of HIV/AIDS: an ethical imperative. *Journal of the Royal Society of Medicine.* **93**: 453–6.

Blair I (1999) Personal communication. Telephone conversation with author, 9 April.

Boriello P (2000) *The Re-emergence of Diphtheria and Concerted European Response.* Presentation at International Conference on Emerging, Re-emerging and Drug-Resistant Infections in Central and Eastern Europe on 28 March 2000 at the National Institute of Hygiene, Warsaw.

Bourdelais P and Dodin A (1987) *Visages du Choléra.* Belin, Paris.

Bourhy H, Kissi B, Audry L, *et al.* (1999) Ecology and evolution of rabies virus in Europe. *Journal of General Virology.* **80**: 2545–57.

Bouvet E (1985) Une nouvelle conception de la surveillance des maladies transmissibles? *Bulletin Epidémiologique Hebdomadaire.* **20**: 1–2.

Brockington F (1967) *World Health (2e).* J and A Churchill Ltd, London.

Bryant G and Monk P (2001) Final report of the investigation into the North Leicestershire cluster of variant Creutzfeld-Jacob disease. Leicestershire Health Authority, Leicester.

Cairns W and McKeon R (1995) *Introduction to French Law.* Cavendish Publishing Limited, London.

Cassar P (1964) *Medical History of Malta.* Wellcome Historical Medical Library, London.

Centers for Disease Control and Prevention (1995) *Infectious Disease – a global health threat.* CDC, Atlanta.

Centres for Disease Control and Prevention (1994) *Addressing emerging infectious disease threats. A prevention strategy for the United States.* CDC, Atlanta.

Chauvin P and Valleron A-J (1995) Attitude of French general practitioners to the public health surveillance of communicable diseases. *International Journal of Epidemiology.* **24**: 435–40.

Chorba T, Berkelman RL, Safford SK *et al.* (1989) The reportable diseases. Mandatory reporting of infectious diseases by clinicians. *JAMA.* **262**: 3018–26.

Clark DS and Ansay T (1992) *Introduction to the Law of the United States.* Kluwer Law and Taxation Publishers, Deventer, Boston.

Clarkson L (1975) *Death, Disease and Famine in Pre-industrial England.* Gill and Macmillan Ltd, Dublin.

Code général des collectivités territoriales (1997) Berger-Levrault, Paris.

Compton's Interactive Encyclopedia (1996) SoftKey Multimedia Inc.

Darbyshire JH (1995) Tuberculosis: old reasons for a new increase? *BMJ.* **310**: 954–5.

Dedushaj, Jorgensen TR, Leiftucht A *et al.* (2000) *An Outbreak of Tularemia in Kosovo.* Presentation at Fifth EPIET Scientific Seminar on 21 October at the Fondation Mérieux, Veyrier-du-Lac.

Department of the Environment/Department of Health HSG (93)56 (1993) *Public Health: responsibilities of the NHS and the roles of others*. DoE/DoH, London, 24 November.

Department of Health (1996) *Immunisation against Infectious Disease*. HMSO, London.

Department of Health (2001) *Shifting the Balance of Power within the NHS: securing delivery*. Department of Health, London.

Department of Health (2002) *Getting Ahead of the Curve: a strategy for combating infectious diseases (including other aspects of health protection)*. Department of Health, London.

Department of Health and Social Security (1970) *The Future Structure of the National Health Service*. HMSO, London.

Department of Health and Social Security (1974) *Committee of Enquiry Report on the Smallpox Outbreak in London in March and April 1973 (The Cox Report)*. HMSO, London.

Department of Health and Social Security (1986) *The Report of the Committee of Inquiry into an Outbreak of Food Poisoning at Stanley Royd Hospital*. HMSO, London.

Desenclos J-C (1998a) Personal communication. Interview with author, 30 July, Réseau National de Santé Publique, Paris.

Desenclos J-C (1998b) Personal communication. Corrected draft to author, dated 10 September.

Desenclos J-C (2001) Personal communication. Corrected draft to author, dated 29 November.

Detels R and Breslow L (1991) Current scope and concerns in public health. In: WW Holland, R Detels and G Knox (eds) *Oxford Textbook of Public Health* (2e). Oxford University Press, Oxford.

De Valk H (2002) Personal communication. E-mail to author dated 15 May.

Donnelly CA and Ferguson NM (1999) *Statistical Aspects of BSE and vCJD: models for an epidemic*. Chapman & Hall CRC, Boca Raton (Florida), London, New York, Washington DC.

Dubin MD (1995) The League of Nations' Health Organisation. In: PJ Weindling (ed.) *International Health Organisations and Movements 1918–1939*. Cambridge University Press, Cambridge.

Ecole Nationale de Santé Publique (1995) *Santé Publique et Territoires: 10 ans de décentralisation*. Rennes.

Ecole Nationale de Santé Publique (1997) *Le Métier de Médecin Inspecteur de Santé Publique et la Formation*. Rennes.

Elimu (2001) *schools step up aids fight*. elimu update january.

Epidemiological Surveillance Division (ESD) (2001) *Case Definitions and Action Thresholds for Integrated Disease Surveillance (IDS)*. Ministry of Health, Kampala.

Euvax project report (2001) *Scientific and Technical Evaluation of Vaccination Programmes in the European Union*. PSR Consulting Ltd, Helsinki.

Falzon D (1998a) Personal communication. Letter to author, dated 19 February.

Falzon D (1998b) Personal communication. Letter to author, with enclosures. dated 30 January.

Falzon D (2002) Personal communication. E-mail to author, dated 29 March.

Farr W (1885) *Vital Statistics. Memorial volume of selections from the reports and writings of William Farr.* NA Humphreys (ed.). Offices of the Sanitary Institute, London.

Federspiel JF (1984) *The Ballad of Typhoid Mary.* André Deutsch Limited, London.

Fee E (1997) The origins and development of public health in the United States. In: WW Holland, R Detels, J McEwen and GS Omenn (eds) *Oxford Textbook of Public Health* (3e). Oxford University Press, Oxford.

Feldman G, Srivastava P, Eden E *et al.* (1997) Detention until cure as a last resort: New York's experience with involuntary in-hospital civil detention of persistently nonadherent tuberculosis patients. *Seminars in Respiratory and Critical Care Medicine.* **18**: 493–501.

Gałązka A (2001) Błonica w Polsce (Diphtheria in Poland). In: J Kostrzewskiego, W Magdzika and D Naruszewicz-Lesiuk (eds) *Choroby zakaźnie i ich ziemiach polskich w XX wieku.* Wydawnictwo Lekarskie PZWL, Warsaw.

Galbraith NS (1977) A national centre for the surveillance and control of communicable disease. *Proceedings of the Royal Society of Medicine, Section of Epidemiology and Community Medicine.* **70**: 889–93.

Galbraith NS (1981) A national public health service. *Journal of the Royal Society of Medicine.* **74**: 16–21.

Galbraith NS (1996) *Port Health Services in Malta: a report to the Chief Government Medical Officer.* Department of Health, Valletta.

Galbraith NS (1998) *CDSC's Origin and Creation.* Oral presentation (recorded on videotape) at Scientific Programme marking 21st Anniversary Celebrations at CDSC, Colindale, London, 11 December.

Gasner MR, Maw KL, Feldman GE *et al.* (1999) The use of legal action in New York City to ensure treatment of tuberculosis. *New England Journal of Medicine.* **340**: 359–65.

Girard J-F (1998) *Quand la Santé devient Publique.* Hachette Littératures, Paris.

Gostin, LO (1986) The future of public health law. *American Journal of Law and Medicine.* **XII**: 461–90.

Graitcer PL and Burton AH (1987) The epidemiologic surveillance project: a computer-based system for disease surveillance. *American Journal of Preventive Medicine.* **3**: 123–7.

Graitcer PL and Thacker SB (1986) The French Connection. *American Journal of Public Health.* **76**: 1285–6.

Graunt J (1662) *Natural and Political Observations upon the Bills of Mortality.* London: Tho: Roycroft, for John Martin, James Allestry and Tho: Dicas.

Grzemska M (2000) *TB Burden and Status of TB Control in Eastern Europe.* Oral presentation at International Conference on Emerging, Re-emerging and Drug-Resistant Infections in Central and Eastern Europe on 28 March at the National Institute of Hygiene, Warsaw.

Guérin N (1996) Evaluation des programmes de vaccination. *Revue d'Epidémiologie et de Santé Publique.* **44**: S73.

Hajjeh RA, Reingold A, Weil A *et al.* (1999) Toxic shock syndrome in the United States: surveillance update, 1979–1996. *Emerging Infectious Diseases.* **5**: 6.

Hamilton G (1998) Personal communication. Letter to author, dated 6 July.

Heine, H (2001). Personal communication. Interview with author, dated 18 October. CDSC, Colindale.

Henderson DA (1999) The looming threat of bioterrorism. Quoted in: LO Gostin (ed.) *Public Health Law and Ethics: a reader*. University of California Press, Berkeley and New York.

Hirst LF (1953) *The Conquest of Plague*. The Clarendon Press, Oxford.

HMSO (1986) First report of the committee of inquiry into the outbreak of Legionnaire's disease in Stafford in April 1985. HMSO, London.

HMSO (1988) Committee of inquiry into the future development of the public health function. *Public Health in England*. HMSO, London.

Holland WW and Stewart S (1997) *Public Health: the vision and the challenge*. The Nuffield Trust, London.

Hubert B *et al.* (1991) La surveillance des maladies transmissibles en France. *Bulletin Epidémiologique Hebdomadaire*. **36**: 155–7.

Hutchins SS and Rosenthal J (1994) Results from WIC Demonstration Projects. Proceedings of the 29th National Immunization Conference, 1994, pp 1–4. US Department of Health and Human Services.

Iliffe J (1998) *East African Doctors*. Cambridge University Press, Cambridge.

Institute of Medicine (1992) *Emerging Infections: microbial threats to health in the United States*. National Academy Press, Washington DC.

Institut de Veille Sanitaire (1999) *Les Vaccinations: actualités et perspectives, Expertise INSERM*. Institut de Veille Sanitaire, Paris.

Institut de Veille Sanitaire (2000) *Mésure de la Couverture Vaccinale en France*. Institut de Veille Sanitaire, Paris.

Ironside J (2001) High vCJD rates in Scotland could be due to poor diet. *BMJ*. **323**: 590.

Kimberlin RH and Walker CA (1989) Pathogenesis of scrapie in mice after intragastric infection. *Virus Research*. **12**: 213–20.

Korycka Maria (2002a) Personal communication. Letter to author, dated 12 January.

Korycka, Maria (2002b) Personal communication. Letter to author, dated 6 August.

Kostrzewski J and Tylewska-Wierzbanowska S (2001) *Dur wysypkowy w Polsce* (Typhus fever in Poland). In: J Kostrzewskiego, W Magdzika and D Naruszewicz-Lesiuk (eds) *Choroby zakaźnie i ich zwalczanie na ziemiach polskich w XX wieku*. Warsaw: Wydawnictwo Lekarskie PZWL.

Lamunu M (2002) Personal communication. Interview with author, Ministry of Health, Kampala, 28 August.

Langmuir AD (1963) The surveillance of communicable diseases of national importance. *New England Journal of Medicine*. **268**: 182–92.

Langmuir AD (1976) William Farr: founder of modern concepts of surveillance. *International Journal of Epidemiology*. **5**: 13–18.

Last JM (ed.) (1983) *A Dictionary of Epidemiology*. Oxford University Press, New York.

Lederberg J (1994) *Addressing Emerging Disease Threats: a preventive strategy for the United States*. Centers for Disease Control and Prevention, Atlanta.

Leviticus *Chapter 13. Verses 45 and 46.*

Lewis J (1991) The origins and development of public health in the UK. In: W Holland, R Detels and G Knox (eds) *Oxford Textbook of Public Health* (2e). Oxford University Press, Oxford.

Lewis, R (2003) Routine childhood immunisation coverage in Uganda. Personal communication. E-mail to author, dated 6 January.

Loudon I (1998) Personal communication. Interview with author. Green College, Oxford, 13 October.

Lubega BM (1997) *A Four-language Easy Communication Pocket Book*: *Luganda, English, KiSwahili, German.* Pan Africa Books, Kampala.

Lwamafa DKW (2002a) Personal communication. Interview with author. Ministry of Health, Kampala, 26 August.

Lwamafa DKW (2002b) Personal communication. File attachment to e-mail to author, dated 12 November.

McGrew RE (1985) *Encyclopedia of Medical History.* Macmillan Press, London.

McKeown T (1979) *The Role of Medicine.* Basil Blackwell, Oxford.

Madsen KM, Hviid A, Vestergaard M *et al.* (2002) A population-based study of measles, mumps and rubella vaccination and autism. *New England Journal of Medicine.* **347**: 1477–82.

Magdzik W (2000a) Personal communication. Interview with author. National Institute of Hygiene, Warsaw, 27 March.

Magdzik W (2000b) *Hepatitis B in Poland, Eastern and Central Europe and the Newly Independent States.* Presentation at International Conference on Emerging, Re-emerging and Drug-Resistant Infections in Central and Eastern Europe on 28 March 2000 at the National Institute of Hygiene, Warsaw.

Magdzik W (2002a) Personal communication. Letter to author, dated 1 February.

Magdzik W (2002b) Personal communication. Letter to author, dated 22 March.

MALTA Information (1995) Department of Information, Valletta.

Mazurek J, Hutin Y, McNutt L-A and Morse DL (2002) Evaluation of hepatitis C surveillance in Poland in 1998. *Epidemiology Infect.* **129**: 119–25.

Mazurek J, Zieliński A and Hutin Y Risk factors for acquisition of hepatitis C virus infection in hospital settings. (In Press)

Mead R (1720) *A Short Discourse Concerning Pestilential Contagion and the Methods to be Used to Prevent it.* Printed for Sam Buckley and Ralph Smith, London.

Meffre C, Aguilera J-F, Hahne S *et al.* (2000) *Invasive Meningococcal Disease Following the Hajj 2000.* Presentation at Fifth EPIET Scientific Seminar on 21 October 2000 at the Fondation Mérieux, Veyrier-du-Lac.

Middleton JD, Binysh K and Pollock GT (1985) Measles – there ought to be a law against it. *Lancet.* **II**: 1180.

Milne LM, Plom A, Strudley I *et al.* (1999) *Escherichia coli* 0157 incident associated with a farm open to members of the public. *Communicable Disease and Public Health.* **2**: 22–6.

Ministère de la Santé Publique (1995) *Guide des Vaccinations.* Paris.

Ministère de la Santé Publique (1999) *Guide des Vaccinations.* Paris.

Ministère de L'Emploi et de la Solidarité (1999) *Guide des Vaccinations.* Paris.

Ministère du Travail et des Affaires Sociales (1996) *La Surveillance des Maladies Transmissibles en France*. Paris.

Ministry of Health (1940) *Memorandum on the Production of Artificial Immunity against Diphtheria*. HMSO, London.

Ministry of Health (1946) *Report of the Chief Medical Officer for the Years 1939– 1945*. HMSO, London.

Ministry of Health (1951) *Report of the Chief Medical Officer for 1948 and 1949*. HMSO, London.

Ministry of Health (1963) *Active Immunisation against Infectious Disease*. HMSO, London.

Ministry of Health (1968) *The Administrative Structure of the Medical and Related Services in England and Wales*. HMSO, London.

Ministry of Health, Uganda (1995) *Burden of Disease Study*. Kampala.

MMWR (1991) *National Electronic Telecommunications System for Surveillance – United States, 1990–1991*. **40**/No. 29: 502–3.

MMWR (2001) *Update: investigation of anthrax associated with intentional exposure and interim public health guidelines*. **50**/No. 41: 889–93.

Monaghan S (2002) *The State of Communicable Disease Law*. The Nuffield Trust for Research and Policy Studies in Health Services, London.

Monin E (1888) *Rapport sur l'Exposition d'Hygiène de Varsovie*. Société des Nations: Organisation d'Hygiène, Paris.

Morelle A (1996) La Défaite de la Santé Publique. Flammarion, Paris.

Morse DL (1993) Personal communication. Interview with author. New York State Department of Health, Albany, NY. 26 November.

Morse DL and DeHovitz J (2000) *Fogarty International Training and Research Opportunities in AIDS/HIV, TB, and Emerging Infections*. New York State Department of Health, Albany, and State University of New York, Brooklyn.

Morse SS (1995) Factors in the emergence of infectious diseases. *Emerging Infectious Diseases*. **1**: 7–15.

Mortimer PP (2001) The OVCD, and what's emerging in England and Wales. *Communicable Disease and Public Health*. **4**: 2–3.

Mullan F (1989) *Plagues and Politics*. Basic Books, Inc, New York.

Muscat M (2001) Personal communication. E-mail to author, dated 18 October.

Myers G, MacInnes K and Korber B (1992) The emergence of simian/human immunodeficiency viruses. *AIDS Res Hum Retroviruses*. **8**: 373–86.

Nahmias AJ *et al.* (1986) Evidence for human infection with an HTLV III/LAV-like virus in central Africa, 1959. *Lancet*. **1**: 1279–80.

National Academy of Science's Institute of Medicine (1992) *Emerging Infections: microbial threats to health in the United States*. National Academy Press, Washington DC.

National Center for Infectious Diseases (1994) *Addressing Emerging Infectious Disease Threats*. CDC Atlanta.

Nicoll A (2001) Personal communication. Corrected draft to author, dated 18 October.

Orenstein WA (1998) Personal communication. Letter to author, with enclosures, dated 5 March.

Orenstein WA, Hinman AR and Rodewald LE (eds) (1999) *Vaccines* (3e). WB Saunders Co., Philadelphia.

Orenstein WA, Hinman AR and Williams WW (1991) *The Impact of Legislation on Immunisation in the United States.* Proceedings of the Second National Immunisation Conference, Public Health Association of Australia, Canberra, 27 May.

Parashar UD, Bresee JS, Gentsch JR *et al.* (1998) Rotavirus. *Emerging Infectious Diseases.* **4**: 561.

Péquignot H (1954) Eléments de politique et d'administration sanitaires. Quoted in: F Brockington (1967) *World Health* (2e). J & A Churchill Ltd, London.

PHLS National Surveillance Group (1997) *A Strategic Framework for Strengthening Communicable Disease in England and Wales 1997–1999.* PHLS, London.

Pollock GT (1992) *Communicable Disease Control in the United States.* Public Health Division, Department of Health, London.

Pollock GT (1993) *'Making London better'* and *Communicable Disease Control.* Thames Regional Health Authorities, London.

Pollock GT (1996) *Some Aspects of Communicable Disease Control in Malta: report to the Chief Government Medical Officer.* Department of Health, Valletta.

Pollock G, Bhopal RS, O'Mahony M and Strangeways J (1991) *The Medical Role in Communicable Disease Control in England: a survey of manpower, responsibilities and training.* Faculty of Public Health Medicine, London.

Poor Law Commissioners (1842) Report from Edwin Chadwick.

Population Information Program (2002) Youth and HIV/AIDS: can we avoid catastrophe? *Population Reports* **Series L**: Number 12. Center for Community Problems, Johns Hopkins University, Baltimore.

Quinlisk P (1998) Personal communication. Letter to author, dated 25 November.

Réseau National de Santé Publique (1996) *Ses Missions et Son Fonctionnement.* Présentation Générale, Paris.

Réseau National de Santé Publique (1997) *Bulletin Épidémiologique Annuel.* Numéro 1.

Rey M (1980) *Vaccinations.* Masson, Paris.

Rosen G (1958) *A History of Public Health.* The Johns Hopkins University Press, Baltimore and London.

Sadkowska-Todys M (2001) Personal communication. Interview with author. National Institute of Hygiene, Warsaw, 11 June.

Salisbury D (1999) Public health and regulatory issues. In: W Orenstein, AR Hinman and LE Rodewald (eds) *Vaccines* (3e). WB Saunders Co, Philadelphia.

Sencer DJ (1995) *The Anatomy, Physiology and Occasional Pathology of the Surveillance System in the United States of America.* WHO, Geneva.

Shelton JD and Johnston B (2001) Condom gap in Africa: evidence from donor agencies and key informants. *BMJ.* **323**: 139.

Smallman-Raynor M and Cliff A (2000) *The Past is Before Us: historical geography of epidemics.* The Wellcome Trust Annual Review 1999/2000.

Smallman-Raynor M, Cliff A and Haggett P (1992) *London International Atlas of AIDS.* Blackwell Reference Series, London.

Smith R (2002) The discomfort of patient power. Editorial, *BMJ.* **324**: 497–8.

Smith R, O'Connell S and Palmer S (2000) Lyme disease surveillance in England and Wales, 1986–1998. *Emerging Infectious Diseases.* **6**: 404–7.

Stern BJ (1927) *Should We Be Vaccinated?* Harper and Bros, New York and London.

Szata W (2000) AIDS i zakażnie HIV w 1998 roku (AIDS and HIV infection in 1998). In: *Przegląd Epidemiologiczny*. Państwowy Zakad Higieny, Warsaw.

Thacker SB (1996) Surveillance. In: MB Gregg (ed.) *Field Epidemiology*. Oxford University Press, Oxford.

Thacker SB and Berkelman RL (1988) Public health surveillance in the United States. *Epidemiologic Reviews*. The Johns Hopkins University School of Hygiene and Public Health. **10**: 165–89.

Thacker SB and Berkelman RL (1992) History of public health surveillance. In: W Halperin and EL Baker (eds) *Public Health Surveillance*. Van Norstrand Reinhold, New York.

Thacker SB and Gregg MB (1996) Implementing the concepts of William Farr: the contributions of Alexander D Langmuir to public health surveillance and communications. *American Journal of Epidemiology*. **144**: S23–S28.

Tocque K (1999) Personal communication. Interview with author at CDSC (West Midlands), 9 April.

Tylewska-Wierzbanowska S and Gałązka A (1998) *The National Institute of Hygiene*. Papirus Ltd, Warsaw.

Updike J (1994) Wildlife. In: *Afterlife*. Knopf, New York.

Valleron A-J, Bouvet E, Garnerin P *et al.* (1986) A computer network for the surveillance of communicable diseases: the French experiment. *American Journal of Public Health*. **76**: 1289–92.

Valleron A-J and Garnerin P (1993) Computerised surveillance of communicable diseases in France. *Communicable Disease Report*. **3 Review No. 6**: R82—R87.

Van Ingen F (2001) Les généalistes sentinelles de santé publique. *Impact Médecin Hebdo*. **530**: 32–3.

Wakefield A, Dhillon AP, Tomson MA *et al.* (1998) Ileal-lymphoid-nodular hyperplasia, non-specific colitis and pervasive developmental disorder in children. *Lancet*. **351**: 637–41.

Walford D and Noah N (1999) Emerging infectious diseases – United Kingdom. *Emerging Infectious Diseases*. **5**: 189–94.

Watson BA (2000) Personal communication. Letter to author, dated 6 November.

Weindling PJ (2000) *Epidemics and Genocide in Eastern Europe 1840–1945*. Oxford University Press, Oxford.

World Health Organization (1991) *Legionnaire's disease – the 1976 outbreak in the United States*. WHO, Geneva.

World Health Organization (2003) *Coronavirus Never Before Seen in Humans is the Cause of SARS* – Update 1, 16 April. WHO, Geneva.

World Health Organization: Uganda Country Office (2001) *Immunisation Drop-out in Uganda*. IDS Health Information Bulletin, September.

WHO/UNICEF (2002) *Review of National Immunization Coverage (Uganda)*, June 2002.

Zalite M (2000) *Epidemiologic Situation of Infectious Diseases in Latvia*. Presentation at International Conference on Emerging, Re-emerging and Drug-Resistant Infections in Central and Eastern Europe on 29 March 2000 at the National Institute of Hygiene, Warsaw.

Index